ecg
arrhythmia interpretation:
a programmed text
for health care personnel

harold a. braun, m.d.
gerald a. diettert, m.d.

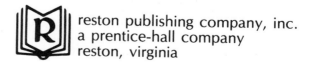
reston publishing company, inc.
a prentice-hall company
reston, virginia

Library of Congress Cataloging in Publication Data

Braun, Harold A
  ECG arrhythmia interpretation.

  Includes index.
    1. Arrhythmia—Diagnosis—Programmed instruction.
  2. Electrocardiography—Programmed instruction.
  I. Diettert, Gerald A., joint author. II. Title.
  [DNLM: 1. Arrhythmia—Programmed texts. 2. Electrocardiography—
  Programmed texts. WG18 B825e]
  RC685.A65B7   616.1'28'0754   78–31496
  ISBN 0–8359–1551–4
  ISBN 0–8359–1550–6 pbk.

© 1979 by Reston Publishing Company, Inc.
A Prentice-Hall Company
Reston, Virginia 22090

10 9 8 7 6 5 4 3 2 1

Printed in the United States of America

contents

introduction

Arrhythmia electrocardiography is difficult enough without having to study it from multiple sources: lecture notes (often written in the dark!), lantern slides, textbooks, and a stack of tracings. Each of these sources is necessary, but we believe your study will be more profitable if guided by material in this programmed text.

HOW TO USE THIS BOOK

Programmed instruction is useful when the material to be covered is too large for detailed presentation in the classroom. It is especially good for self-instruction, the kind of instruction which really sticks. The student who actively participates in the learning experience is the student who remembers best.

Programmed learning provides systematically arranged lumps of knowledge. Each lump or instructional unit is arranged in a "frame." Each frame is a step, each step leads to the next and each is based on previous steps.

Thus you must *do* something with each frame—write out a word or phrase or match items. Some of the frames may appear so simple that you will be tempted to answer them mentally. Don't! Write your answer in the space which is provided.

Don't peek. Use the mask to cover the right hand column until you have written down your response. Don't weaken the learning process by looking back at previous frames. Look back only after you have wrestled with the question and have made some response. If your response was wrong, then go back and see where you went astray.

Thus you should follow four steps with each frame:

1. Read the question.
2. Write down your answer in the space provided.
3. Move the mask covering the answers so that you can check your response. Do not uncover the frames following the one on which you are working.
4. If your answer is right, go on to the next frame. If wrong, correct your mistake and avoid later confusion which would result from a faulty background.

At the close of each chapter is a problem-solving section. Compare your answers with those in the appendix.

STUDY SUGGESTIONS

Before the lecture, complete the assigned section in the text. *During* the lecture, ask the instructor to clear up any uncertainties. *After* the lecture, review the material once more. If you are still confused on some point, come to the next class with questions in hand.

A good ECG calipers will help.

STEPS IN THE USE OF PROGRAMMED MATERIAL

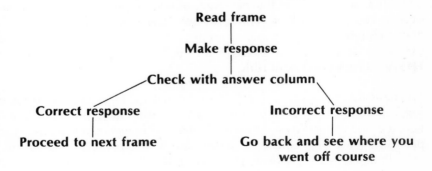

Read frame

Make response

Check with answer column

Correct response

Proceed to next frame

Incorrect response

Go back and see where you went off course

acknowledgements

We are grateful for the help of many people, especially Vera Wills, Barbara Noel, Ethel Staat of the Western Montana Clinic; readers who pointed out areas of confusion; and Drs. Norman Makous, John Gilson, Borys Surawicz, James Gouaux and Richard Weber for helpful criticism.

Electrocardiographic illustrations were obtained from the files of the Western Montana Clinic, and from the Special Care Unit of St. Patrick Hospital, Missoula, Montana.

HB and GD

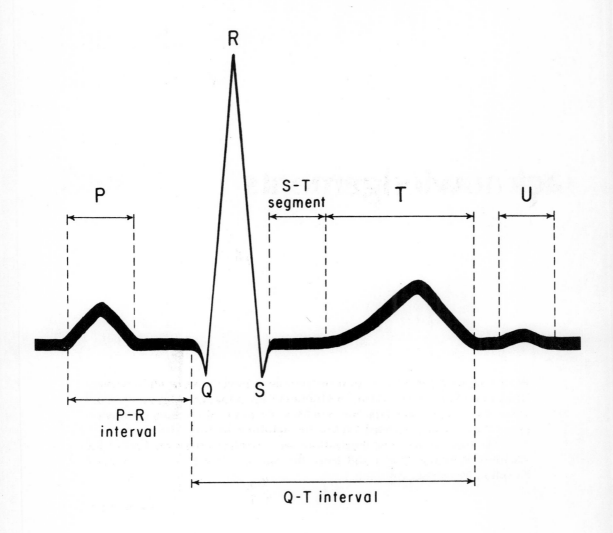

chapter 1

electrical anatomy of the heart

1. Electrical anatomy of the heart.

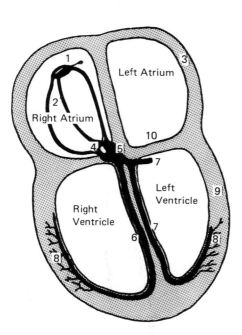

*The term junctional is discussed on page 270.

2. With wonderful reliability, the sinus node periodically releases an electrical impulse which initiates the heart cycle.

3. The normal heart cycle is initiated by an electrical discharge from the

    __✓__ sinus node.

    _____ A-V node.

    _____ ventricles.

    sinus node.

4. We can only infer activity of the sinus node, for its discharge produces no ECG deflection. However, when the sinus node electrical discharge spreads through the atria, the P wave of the ECG is inscribed.

5. In a sinus cycle, there is no ECG evidence that the sinus node has discharged until the depolarization wave reaches the _atria_ and produces the P wave.

    atrial muscle

6. Depolarization means about the same thing as flow of electrical current.
   Depolarization of the sinus node produces no ECG deflection.
   Depolarization of the atria produces the P wave.
   Depolarization of the ventricles produces the QRS complex.

7. The P wave results from current flowing

    _____ in the bundle branches.

    _____ in the ventricles.

    __✓__ in the atria.

    in the atria.

8. P Wave   QRS Complex

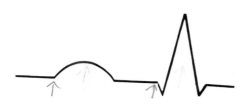

With an arrow, show where the atria were depolarized and where the ventricles were depolarized.

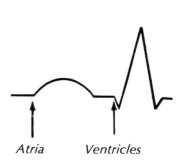

Atria   *Ventricles*

---

9. The atria are joined to the ventricles by fibrous tissue of the A-V groove, a poor conductor. Thus, a special pathway is required to permit conduction of electrical impulses from atria to ventricles. This is the A-V node or A-V junctional apparatus.

---

10. The beginning of the P wave marks the beginning of atrial depolarization. The beginning of the QRS complex marks the beginning of ventricular depolarization. Review the illustration. Between the beginning of P and the beginning of QRS is the

_____ T wave.

___✓__ PR interval.

PR interval.

---

11. During the PR interval the depolarization wave is spreading through the atria, the A-V junctional issue and bundle branches. However, most of the delay between atrial and ventricular activation is due to relatively slow conduction through the junctional tissue (A-V node).

---

12. A long PR interval usually means that disturbance is present in the

_____ ventricles.

_____ sinus node.

___✓__ A-V node.

A-V node.

13. We can only infer activity of the A-V node as well as the sinus node for these structures electrically are silent on the usual ECG. Their depolarization produces no ECG deflection.

14. In a sinus cycle there is no ECG evidence of A-V node activity until the depolarization wave reaches ventricular muscle and produces the _QRS_____.

QRS complex.

15.

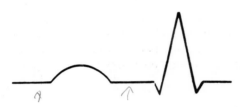

With an arrow, show where the sinus node might have discharged and where the A-V node might have depolarized.

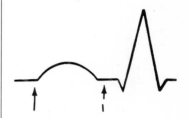

Sinus   A-V
node   node

16. From the A-V junction, the depolarization wave flows down the bundle of His and the bundle branches.

Finally, the Purkinje fibers (small divisions of the bundle branches) carry the depolarization wave to the ventricular muscle fibers. Depolarization of the ventricular muscle produces the QRS complex.

17. The QRS complex begins when the impulse reaches the

_____ bundle of His.

__✓__ ventricular muscle.

_____ A-V node.

ventricular muscle.

18. Number the following structures in the order of their activation during a normal sinus cycle.

_5_ bundle branches

_3_ A-V node

_1_ sinus node

_7_ ventricular muscle

_2_ atrial muscle

_4_ bundle of His

_6_ Purkinje fibers

_2_ internodal and sino-atrial tracts

1—sinus node

2—internodal and sino-atrial tracts

3—atrial muscle

4—A-V node

5—bundle of His

6—bundle branches

7—Purkinje fibers

8—ventricular muscle

---

19. The specialized conduction apparatus within the ventricles is called the His-Purkinje system. Fibers of the His-Purkinje system are similar to the transmission lines of an electrical system. They distribute the stimulation wave throughout the ventricles and do so at high speed—4000 mm. per sec.

---

20. A normal duration (narrow) QRS indicates that the impulse has been distributed via the rapidly-conducting His-Purkinje system.

---

21. Rapid distribution of the depolarization wave through the ventricles will produce a QRS which is

___ narrow.

___ broad.

narrow.

---

22. A narrow (normal duration) QRS indicates that distribution of the impulse through the ventricles has been

___ rapid.

___ slow.

rapid.

23.

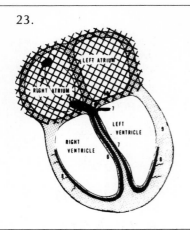

IMPULSES OF SUPRAVENTRICULAR ORIGIN CAN UTILIZE THE HIS-PUR-KINJE SYSTEM

The His-Purkinje system is utilized fully only if the depolarization wave comes down from above—from a supraventricular origin.

24. Generally, the His-Purkinje system can be utilized only by depolarization waves which arise in the sinus node, atria, or A-V junctional tissue (supraventricular cycles). Thus, only cycles of supraventricular origin produce narrow QRS complexes.

25. If QRS duration is normal, we can conclude that the initiating impulse arose in a

_____ ventricular focus.

__✓__ supraventricular focus.

supraventricular focus. (Only supraventricular cycles utilize the high speed transmission system.)

26. Ordinary myocardial fibers conduct slowly—500 mm. per sec. If the ordinary ventricular muscle fibers must be relied upon to conduct the depolarization wave, the resulting QRS complex will be broad. Ordinary muscle fibers must be used for ventricular spread of the depolarization wave in two circumstances:

1. Dysfunction in the His-Purkinje system.

2. Ventricular origin of the depolarization wave.

27. A broad QRS indicates

_____ rapid

_✓_ slow

slow

transmission of the depolarization wave
through the ventricles.

28. Slow distribution of the depolarization wave throughout the ventricles is
indicated by a broad QRS. Slow distribution may occur for two reasons:

1. Although the cycle is of supraventricular origin, an ailing His-Purkinje
system conducts it slowly. Bundle branch block is one of the causes of
a broad QRS of supraventricular origin.

2. A depolarization wave of ventricular origin cannot utilize the His-Purkinje system. Distribution must occur via slowly conducting, ordinary
muscle fibers. A ventricular premature complex (initiated by an impulse
arising in the ventricles) is one of the causes of a broad QRS of ventricular origin.

SUMMARY—CHAPTER I

1. Normally, heart rate and rhythm are under control of the sinus node.

2. The electrical stimulus released from the SA node is distributed via specialized conduction tissues, of which the most important are the A-V node, the bundles, and their divisions.

3. As the stimulus depolarizes the atria, the P wave is produced. There is some delay getting through the A-V junctional apparatus; the PR interval results.

4. Eventually the depolarization wave spreads through the His-Purkinje system to the ventricular muscle fibers, producing the QRS complex.

5. Because the His-Purkinje system transmits rapidly, QRS normally is narrow.

6. If the His-Purkinje system is ailing, ventricular spread may be slow and QRS will be broad. The second cause of a broad QRS is ventricular origin of the cycle. If so, transmission must occur via ordinary heart muscle, a slow conductor.

PROBLEMS—CHAPTER I

Normally the heart cycle is under control of the (1) _S. A. node_. The stimulus released from the sinus node is distributed by specialized conduction tissues, of which the most important are the A-V junction, the right bundle branch, the left bundle branch, and its fascicles.

As the depolarization wave activates the atria, the (2) _P_ wave is produced. There is some delay in transmission through the A-V junctional apparatus; the (3) _P-R_ interval results. Finally, ventricular muscle fibers are depolarized; the (4) _QRS complex_ results. Because the His-Purkinje system transmits rapidly, all the ventricular muscle normally is activated within a very short time. Therefore, the normal QRS complex is narrow.

If the His-Purkinje system is ailing, ventricular activation will require more time and QRS will be (5) _____ (narrow) _✓_ (broad). Another cause of a broad QRS is ventricular origin of the cycle.

chapter 2

the ecg waves

1. A telegram is a piece of paper with a record on it. A telegraph is an instrument. An electrocardiograph is

    ____✓ an instrument.

    _____ a piece of paper.

    an instrument.

2. TERMINOLOGY: The electrocardiogram (ECG) is a written record of the electrical activity of the heart. The major waves or deflections of an ECG cycle traditionally are labeled P, QRS, and T. The P wave represents depolarization (electrical discharge) of the atria. The QRS complex represents depolarization of the ventricles. The T wave represents repolarization (electrical recharging) of the ventricles. The ST segment is that portion of the tracing between the end of QRS and the beginning of the T wave.

TERMINOLOGY OF THE ELECTROCARDIOGRAM

3.

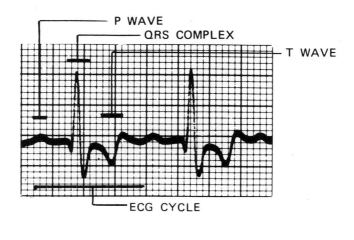

P WAVE
QRS COMPLEX
T WAVE
ECG CYCLE

4.

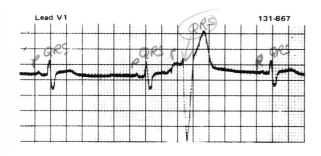

Lead V1   131-867

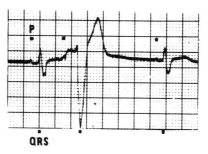

P

QRS

Label the P waves and QRS complexes in this rhythm strip.

5. The QRS complex represents electrical discharge of the

_____ atria.

✓ ventricles.

ventricles.

6. Depolarization is a term given to the process in which a muscle cell loses the electrical charge normally present across its membrane.

   Thus, in frame 5, "electrical discharge of the ventricles" also might be written "depolarization of the ventricles."

---

7. A positive deflection in a QRS complex always is an R wave. A negative deflection may be a Q wave or an S wave.

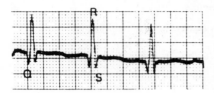

Q (negative deflection which precedes R)

R (positive deflection)

S (negative deflection which follows R)

VARIOUS QRS COMPLEXES

8.

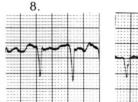 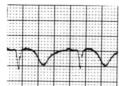 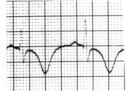 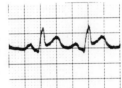

The waves due to ventricular depolarization customarily are called the QRS complex, even though this consists of only one or two deflections. The QRS complex may be totally negative and then is termed a QS deflection (frame 11, strip A). It may have only an R wave (frame 14) or an RS (frame 9, lead VI).

9.

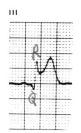 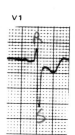 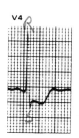 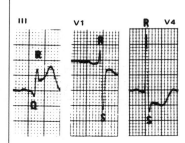

Label the deflections in these QRS complexes. Each has an R wave but only one has a Q wave.

10.

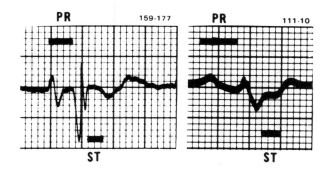

In addition to the major deflections of the ECG cycle, you will be dealing with the **PR interval** and **ST segment.**

The PR interval extends from the onset of the P wave to the beginning of the QRS complex, whether QRS begins with an R or a Q wave.

11.

QS

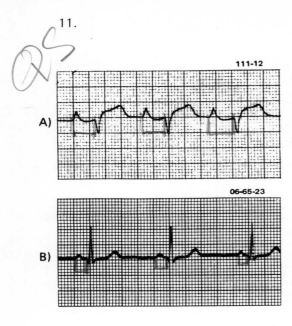

111-12

A)

06-65-23

B)

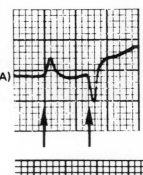

A)

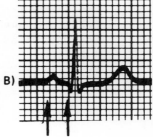

B)

Indicate beginning and end of the PR interval.

In strip A, note that QRS consists only of a negative deflection. Such a form is termed a QS wave.

12. The ST segment commences at the end of QRS complex and terminates at the beginning of the _____.

QRS
T wave.

13. Normally the ST segment is neither elevated nor depressed. Heart muscle injury is a common cause of ST segment displacement.

14.

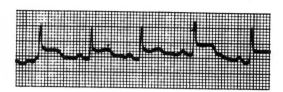

This record was obtained soon after myocardial infarction. The ST segment is _____.

elevated.

15. The T wave usually is the last large deflection in the cycle. However, a small wave may follow T.

What name would you choose for a wave which comes after P, Q, R, S, and T?

_____

U wave

16.

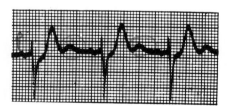

Label the U waves.

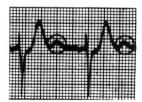

SUMMARY—CHAPTER II

1. The electrocardiograph is an instrument. The electrocardiogram is a written record of the electrical activity of the heart.

2. Depolarization and electrical discharge have similar meanings.

3. The P wave represents depolarization of the atria.

4. QRS represents depolarization of the ventricles. The QRS complex may consist of a QS deflection, only an R wave or an RS.

5. The PR interval extends from the beginning of the P wave to the beginning of the QRS complex.

6. Between the end of QRS and the beginning of T is the ST segment.

7. The T wave represents repolarization of the ventricles.

PROBLEMS—CHAPTER II

1. In these cycles, label P, Q, R, S, and T.

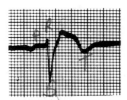 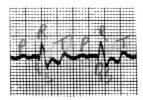

2. The PR interval is measured from the beginning of the P wave to
   beginning - QRS

3. The ST segment extends from the end of QRS to the beginning of the T
   wave.

4. These are tough arrhythmias. Label the QRS complexes. Note the different shape in different people.

Label the P waves if you can. Note the following:

1. P waves are not always visible.
2. A P wave does not necessarily precede each QRS.
3. Appearance varies in different people and in different electrical hook-ups (leads), shown here as Mon. (II) or MCL-1.

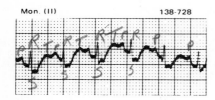

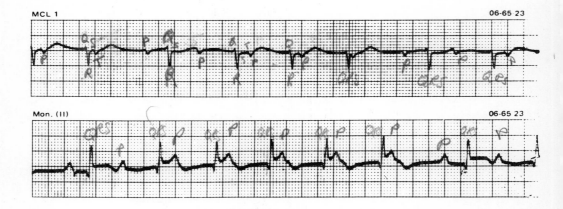

chapter 3

measurements of amplitude and time

1.

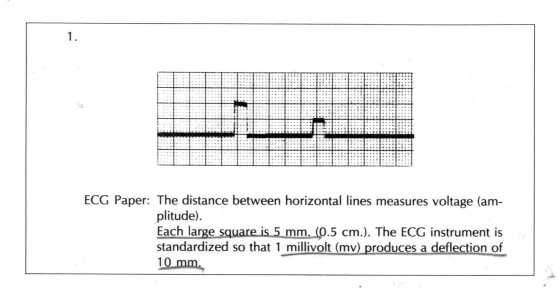

ECG Paper: The distance between horizontal lines measures voltage (amplitude).
Each large square is 5 mm. (0.5 cm.). The ECG instrument is standardized so that 1 millivolt (mv) produces a deflection of 10 mm.

2.

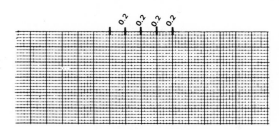

ECG Paper: The distance between vertical lines measures time.
The time between two fine vertical lines is 0.04 sec.

3. One big square contains five 0.04 sec. squares and represents

✓ _____ 0.20 sec.   _____ 1.0 sec.

_____ 5.0 sec.

0.20 sec.

4.

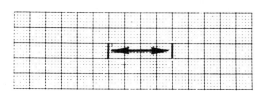

The time interval indicated by the arrow is 0.8 sec.

0.80 sec.

5. How many 0.04 sec. squares are present in 60 seconds?

1500

$$\frac{1500}{0.04\overline{)60.00}}$$

6. If the rhythm is regular, rate equals 1500 divided by

the number of 0.04 sec. squares between two complexes.

TABLE FOR CALCULATION OF HEART RATE

(if rhythm is regular)

Cycle Length (sec.)	Number of 0.04 sec. squares	Rate	Cycle Length (sec.)	Number of 0.04 sec. squares	Rate
0.16	4	375	0.84	21	72
0.20	5	300	0.88	22	68
			0.92	23	65
0.24	6	250	0.96	24	63
0.28	7	214	1.00	25	60
0.32	8	188	1.04	26	58
0.36	9	168	1.12	28	54
0.40	10	150	1.20	30	50
0.44	11	136	1.28	32	47
0.48	12	125	1.36	34	44
			1.44	36	42
0.52	13	115	1.52	38	40
0.56	14	107			
0.60	15	100	1.60	40	38
			1.68	42	36
0.64	16	94	1.76	44	35
0.68	17	88			
			1.92	48	31
0.72	18	83	2.00	50	30
0.76	19	79			
0.80	20	75			

7.

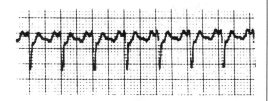

In this tracing, the ventricular rate is about ___150___ /minute.

150
Explanation: There are 10 small squares between QRS complexes. 1500 divided by 10 equals 150.

8. How many 0.20 sec. squares are present in 60 seconds?

_____300_____

$$0.20\overline{)60.00}^{\,300}$$

9. If the rhythm is regular, rate equals 300 divided by

 # - 0.2 sec. squares
÷ 2 complexes

the number of 0.20 sec. squares between two complexes.

10.

Is the rhythm nearly regular?

yes

Yes

How many 0.20 sec. squares are present between cycles? _____3_____

3

What is the heart rate? _____100_____ /min.

$$3\overline{)300}^{\,100}$$

11. The easiest and most accurate way to determine the heart rate is to count the number of cycles in 6 seconds and multiply by 10. If the rhythm is irregular this is the only satisfactory way to determine rate.

12. Rate equals number of complexes in 6 sec. multiplied by _____10_____ .

10

13. One cm. represents ten 0.04 sec. squares.

Fifteen cm. represents _____6_____ sec.

6 sec.
Explanation:
15 × 0.4 sec. = 6 sec.

14. Heart rate equals the number of complexes in 15 cm. (6 sec.) times _____10_____ .

10

15. Time lines usually are printed at the top
of ECG paper, indicating one second or
three second intervals.

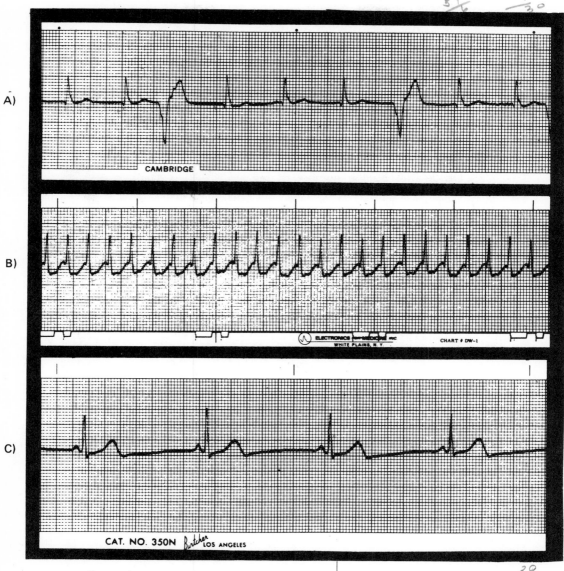

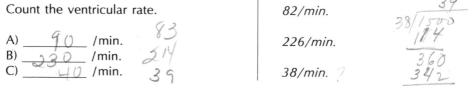

Count the ventricular rate.

A) _____90_____ /min.

B) _____230_____ /min.

C) _____40_____ /min.

82/min.

226/min.

38/min.

16. Heart rate may be counted in several ways:

A) Rhythm regular or irregular:
   Count the number of cycles in 6 sec. and multiply

   × ___*10*___ .

   10

B) Rhythm regular:
   Divide ___*1500*___ by the number of small squares between two cycles.

   1500

C) Rhythm regular:
   Divide 300 by the number of big squares between two cycles.

No. of big squares between 2 cycles	Rate
2	*150*
3	*100*
4	*75*
5	*60*
6	*50*

No. of big squares	Rate
2	*150*
3	*100*
4	*75*
5	*60*
6	*50*

THE PR INTERVAL

17. The PR interval reflects the time required for a depolarization wave to spread from atria to ventricles. Most of the delay is in the region of the A-V node.

    Normally the PR interval is 0.12-0.20 sec. A **long PR** (0.21 sec. or more) suggests delay in the A-V junction.

    A **short PR** (0.11 sec. or less) suggests genesis of the P wave from a focus near or in the A-V node. There are several other causes of a short PR:

    1. Accelerated conduction in the junctional tissue.

    2. Use of accessory A-V conduction pathways which by-pass the region of hold-up in the A-V node.

    3. Sino-atrial block (delayed spread of the excitation wave from sinus node to atrium) with unimpaired internodal conduction.

18.

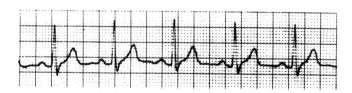

From the beginning of P to the beginning of QRS there are about _____ small squares.

four

Each small square is ___0 04___ sec.

0.04

The PR interval is ___0.16___ sec.

0.16

19.

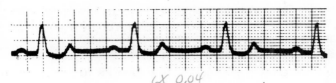

What is the PR interval?   *6× 0.04*   0.24 | 0.24 sec.

What is the heart rate?   54 | 52

A long PR interval usually means abnormality of the

✓ A-V node.

_____ SA node | A-V node.

20. A long PR interval indicates abnormally slow

✓ atrio-ventricular conduction.

_____ intraventricular conduction. | atrio-ventricular conduction.

21. The PR interval begins with the onset of the P wave. This point may be obscured in the prior T wave.

Mon. (II)   **MCL-1**

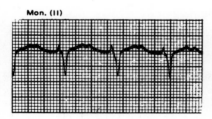   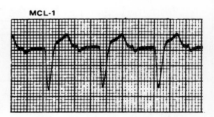

The PR interval ends whenever the QRS complex starts. Traditionally, this interval is called PR even though it may end with a Q rather than an R wave. (See lead MCL-1, above.)

QRS DURATION

22. Remember that a normal impulse utilizes the high speed transmission lines of the His-Purkinje system for rapid activation of the ventricles. A normal duration, narrow QRS means that the His-Purkinje system has been utilized. Impulses of supraventricular origin utilize the His-Purkinje system. If the focus responsible for QRS is in the ventricular muscle, the His-Purkinje system cannot be utilized in normal fashion. Spread throughout the ventricles will be slow. QRS will be broad. QRS also is broad if an impulse of supraventricular origin finds conduction in the His-Purkinje system slow or blocked.

23. Normally the QRS duration in a monitoring lead is 0.10 sec. or less.

24. Each small square is 0.04 sec. or less. Normally the QRS will occupy less than ____3____ small squares.	2 ½

25.

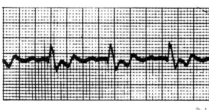

4X.04

What is the QRS duration? 0.16 sec.

0.16 sec.

This QRS is

_____ narrow.

__✓__ broad.

broad.

26.

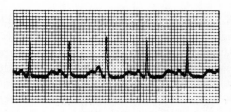

What is the QRS duration?

_0.4⁺_ sec.

This QRS is

✓_____ narrow.

_____ broad.

0.05 sec.

narrow.

SUMMARY—CHAPTER III

1. PR interval is measured from onset of P to onset of QRS. This is true even though QRS begins with a Q wave.

2. Normally, PR interval is 0.12–0.20 sec. A long PR usually is due to delayed conduction in the A-V junction.

3. Normally, QRS duration is 0.10 sec. or less. A broad QRS indicates either:

    1. Delayed conduction (block) of a supraventricular impulse in the His-Purkinje system, or
    2. Origin of the depolarization wave within the ventricles.

4. Heart rate may be determined from the ECG in several ways.

    1. Use the table on page 21 (accurate only if the rhythm is regular).
    2. Divide 1500 by the number of 0.04 sec. squares between two complexes (accurate only if the rhythm is regular).
    3. Divide 300 by the number of 0.20 sec. squares between two complexes (accurate only if the rhythm is regular).

No. of 0.20 sec. squares between two complexes	Rate
1	300
2	150
3	100
4	75
5	60
6	50

    4. Count the number of cycles in six seconds (15 cm.) and multiply by 10.

PROBLEMS—CHAPTER III

1. The easiest and most accurate way to count heart rate is to count the number of cycles in six seconds and multiply by ___*10*___.

2. How many 0.20 sec. squares are present in 60 seconds?   *300*

3. Normally the PR interval is between ___*0.12*___ and ___*0.20*___ sec.

4. Normally the QRS duration in a monitoring lead is ___*0.10*___ sec. or less.

5.

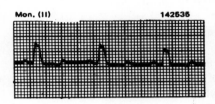

   What is the heart rate?   ___*75*___ /min.

   What is the PR interval?   ___*0.12*___ sec.   *0.14*

   What is the QRS duration?   ___*0.16*___ sec.   *0.11*

6. If the rhythm is regular, rate equals 300 divided by ___*0.20 squares*___.   *x cycles*

   230 (208)

7. What is the heart rate?

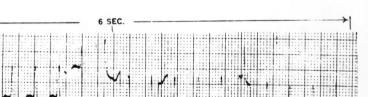

   230

chapter 4

leads and other ecg fundamentals

1. Normally, the heart cycle is initiated by a stimulus released from the

   _____ A-V junction.

   __✓__ sinus node.

   _____ bundle of His.

   sinus node.

2. The stimulus causes cells near the sinus node to change from their resting (polarized) state to an excited (depolarized) condition.

THREE ADJACENT MYOCARDIAL CELLS

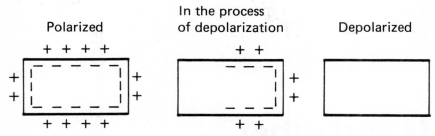

| Polarized | In the process of depolarization | Depolarized |

The depolarization wave sweeps from cell to cell and initiates muscle contraction.

3.

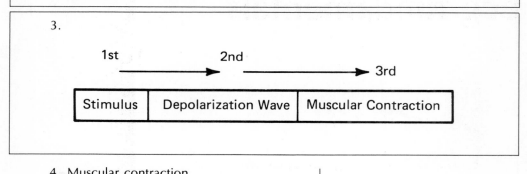

1st ——→ 2nd ——————→ 3rd

| Stimulus | Depolarization Wave | Muscular Contraction |

4. Muscular contraction

_____✓_____ follows depolarization wave.

_____ precedes depolarization wave.

follows depolarization wave.

5. An electrode is a device by which electrical recording apparatus (such as an oscilloscope or electrocardiograph) makes contact with the object from which measurements are to be made. A galvanometer is a meter which measures the voltage difference between two electrodes. An electrocardiograph is a special sort of galvanometer which makes a written record of voltage difference between two electrodes.

Galvanometer

Electrodes

6.

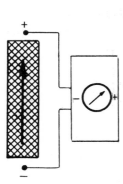

In the diagram, the electrodes of a galvanometer are placed at opposite ends of the myocardial strip. The galvanometer is manufactured in such a way that it shows a positive reading when the depolarization wave is flowing toward the positive electrode.

7.

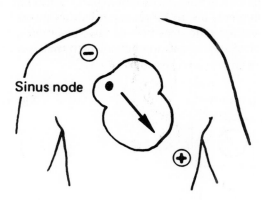

In the diagram, the negative electrode is placed in the vicinity of the right shoulder, at the headward end of the heart. The positive electrode is below the heart and to the left.

Note that the sinus node is at the head end of the atria. Atrial depolarization commencing in the sinus node will move in a footward direction, toward the positive electrode.

Likewise, the greater mass of the ventricles is oriented downward and toward the left. Therefore, one might expect ventricular depolarization in general to move in a direction from head to foot and from right to left. With this electrode placement (so-called monitoring lead II) it is moving toward the positive electrode.

By tradition, the oscilloscope and electrocardiograph are manufactured in such a way that they show a positive wave when the depolarization wave is flowing towards the positive electrode.

8. The galvanometer reading is negative when the depolarization wave

_____ approaches the positive electrode.

_____ moves away from the positive electrode.

moves away from the positive electrode.

9. Since the ECG wave is positive when the depolarization wave is moving towards the positive electrode, negative when the depolarization wave is moving away from the positive electrode, it is not surprising that the deflection will be very small or absent when depolarization is perpendicular to the lead axis (an imaginary line connecting the two electrodes).

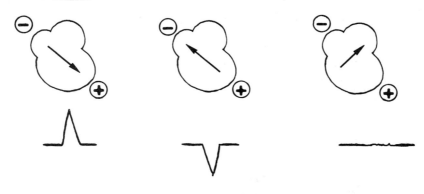

LEAD AXIS

10. **Lead axis** refers to an imaginary line connecting the recording electrodes.

ECG LEADS

11. When a standard electrocardiogram is to be recorded, electrodes are placed on the extremities, as well as on the chest. A switch (**lead selector switch**) then selects the particular electrodes which actually are used to record the desired lead.

An **ECG lead** refers to the connection between the instrument and the body. For example, lead I of a standard ECG refers to a connection with the RA and LA electrodes. In this lead, LA is positive. Thus when current flow is from right to left, lead I will show a positive deflection.

Another example. With lead II, the connection is between the instrument and electrodes on the LL and RA; the LL electrode is positive.

For other leads, the switch selects other electrodes, arranging matters so the proper one is positive.

12.

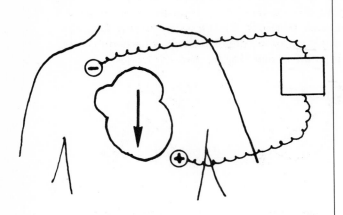

Assume that the arrow indicates the average direction of the depolarization waves through the ventricles. The ECG will record a QRS complex which is chiefly

_____ ✓ positive.

_____ negative.

positive.

13. The **unipolar limb leads** are special modifications of leads I, II, and III. They are called:

aVR—recording from the right arm

aVL—recording from the left arm

aVF—recording from the left foot
(actually from the left leg)

14.

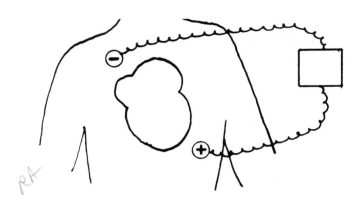

RA

LL

This is the connection for a common monitoring lead, often called "Monitoring Lead II" because its lead axis is similar to that of lead II in the 12-lead ECG.

monitoring lead

15. The lead axis in Mon. II is

✓

_____ from right to left.   *from head to foot.*

✓ _____ from head to foot.   *from right to left.*

_____ from front to back.

16. The lead axis in the sketch, frame 14, is similar to the axis of lead II. *LL + RA*
    +   −

    Lead II records a positive wave when the depolarization wave flows from

    ✓ _____ head to foot.

    _____ foot to head.   *head to foot.*

17.

The depolarization wave is indicated by an arrow.

Will the oscilloscope show a positive, negative or zero voltage when using the monitoring lead (Mon. II)?

pos

Positive

Will the ECG show a positive, negative or zero voltage when the lead selector switch is set at lead II? _pos_

Positive

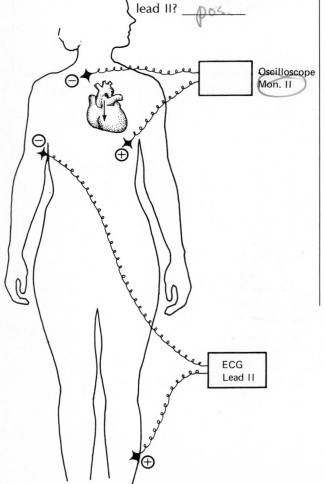

Oscilloscope
Mon. II

ECG
Lead II

18.

The unipolar V leads are recorded from various positions on the chest wall.

The V1 position is in the 4th intercostal space at the right sternal border.

---

19. To record lead V1 the electrode is located in the _____ interspace, just to the

    _____ right

    _____ left

of the sternum.

4th

right

MODIFIED CHEST LEAD-1

20. A useful monitoring lead places the positive electrode in the V1 position, negative electrode at the left shoulder. This is termed MCL-1. The special value of this modified chest lead is its presentation of QRS features. It may or may not be best for P-wave demonstration.

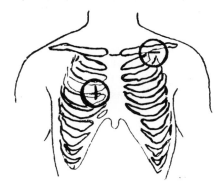

21. The appearance of an object depends upon the shape of the object and upon the point of view.

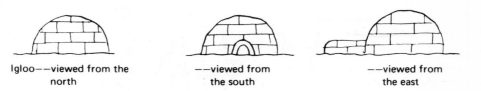

Igloo—viewed from the
north

—viewed from
the south

—viewed from
the east

The lead axis is the point of view used to observe the depolarization wave.

The ECG deflection depends upon the "shape" of the depolarization wave and upon the lead axis.

22.

Mon. (II)

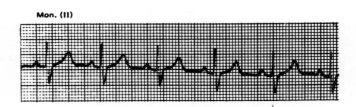

This record was obtained from a monitoring lead with an axis similar to that of lead II. The positive electrode was in the left axilla. The negative electrode was at the right shoulder.

In this patient, the general direction of atrial depolarization was

___✓___ from head to foot.

_____ from foot to head.

from head to foot.

23.

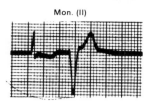

Mon. (II)

This record was obtained from a monitoring lead with an axis similar to that of lead II.

For the first QRS, direction of ventricular depolarization was

✓ _____ from head to foot.

_____ from foot to head.

from head to foot.

For the second complex, the direction of ventricular depolarization was

_____ from head to foot.

✓ _____ from foot to head.

from foot to head.

24. The sinus node is at the head end of the atria.

The sinus node is to the right of the bulk of the atrial muscle.

25. Indicate the direction of the normal atrial depolarization wave.

✓ _____ from right to left

_____ from foot to head

✓ _____ from head to foot

_____ from left to right

from right to left AND from head to foot

26. Because the left ventricular muscle is larger than the right, the sum of the depolarization waves flowing through the ventricular muscle fibers is from right to left.

27. If you want a monitoring lead which will provide a QRS of good amplitude and an upright P wave, you could locate the positive electrode

    _____ below and to the right.

    ✓ below and to the left.

    _____ above and to the right.

    _____ above and to the left.

    below and to the left.

HOW TO RECORD P WAVES

28. To study an arrhythmia, P waves should not be obscured by other portions of the ECG cycle. A 12-lead record often is necessary to find the best "point of view."

    Sometimes a P wave is larger and easier to find in V1 than in the monitoring lead with an axis similar to that of lead II. The chest electrode could be placed anywhere on the chest, looking for a spot where P waves are prominent.

    The V lead wire can be attached to an electrode in the esophagus. Proximity of the esophageal electrode to the atria provides P waves of large amplitude. Alternately, the V lead wire can be attached to the electrode of a pacing catheter which is advanced into the right atrium.

29.

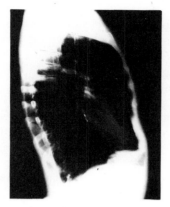

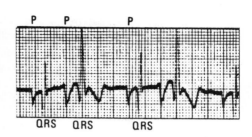

The esophageal electrode was positioned at the left atrial level to record _____ waves of large amplitude.

P waves

30.

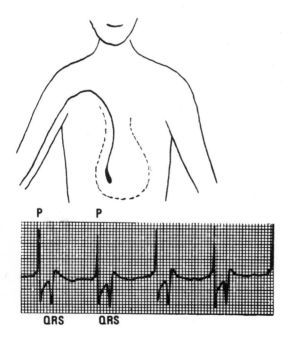

The catheter electrode was advanced from an arm vein into the right atrium. The P wave is huge because the electrode _____ .

is in the atrium.

SUMMARY—CHAPTER IV

1. Stimulation causes a resting cell to lose the electrical charge normally present across its membrane. This process moves down the length of the cell and then to neighboring cells.

2. Depolarization describes this wave-like electrical change.

3. Depolarization induces muscle contraction.

4. Electrode location determines lead axis.

5. The shape of an ECG deflection is determined by the relation between lead axis and the direction of the depolarization wave.

6. Monitoring lead II may be best for study of P waves. Monitoring lead MCL-1 is most popular for study of QRS configuration.

PROBLEMS—CHAPTER IV

1. An ECG deflection will be positive in a given lead if the depolarization wave moves *(toward)* *(away from)* the positive electrode of that lead. The same depolarization wave may produce quite a different deflection in different leads, much as an object may vary in appearance, depending on one's point of observation.

2. The ECG deflection is largest if the lead axis is parallel to the direction of the depolarization wave. The ECG deflection is smallest if the lead axis is perpendic to the direction of the depolarization wave.

3. Another factor determines the size of the deflection. This is the closeness (proximity) of one of the electrodes to the heart. If an exploring electrode is inside the right atrium, the record is called a **right atrial electrogram** and the _____P_____ wave is large.

4. In lead II, the negative electrode is on the right arm and the positive electrode is on the *(left arm)* *(left leg)*.

5. In a monitoring lead with an axis similar to lead II, the P wave normally is *(positive)* *(negative)*.

6. This is true because atrial depolarization starts at the sinus node and spreads *(downward and to the left)* *(upward and to the right)*.

chapter 5

a systematic approach to the rhythm strip

1. An expert horse-trader can size up a steed with a quick glance. But the wise amateur will have a list of points to evaluate systematically before he buys.

2. Systematic evaluation of the ECG

   ☑ ___ is wise.

   ☑ ___ helps to avoid overlooking important features.

   Both answers are correct.

3. PROCEDURE FOR SYSTEMATIC EVALUATION OF A RHYTHM STRIP

Technique
Identify artifact such as alternating current interference, muscle tremor or wandering baseline.

Identify the QRS Complexes
Ventricular rate
QRS duration
Do all complexes have the same configuration?
Ventricular rhythm
    Are there premature QRS complexes?

☐ broad and "different"	☐ narrow and same as
☐ not preceded by	dominant QRS
premature P	☐ preceded by premature P
☐ do not interrupt rhythm	☐ interrupt rhythm of the
of the sinus node	sinus node

Identify the Atrial Complexes
Atrial rate
    Especially when tachycardia or bradycardia is present, it is a good principle to ask: "Could another P wave be hidden halfway between the obvious ones?"
Atrial rhythm
Are there premature P waves?

Evaluate A-V Conduction
PR interval
    Is the PR interval normal (0.12–0.20 sec)?
    Is the PR interval constant?
Is each P wave followed by a QRS complex?

CONCLUSION
Using the above approach, a *description* can be provided, even though an arrhythmia *diagnosis* may not be possible.

ARTIFACTS

4. An artifact is a feature of the ECG record which is not a natural occurrence but is caused by the technique of the recording.

   Artifacts can be recognized easily after you have seen more tracings. The most common artifacts are:

   1. Alternating current (A.C.) interference—regular deflections at 60 cycles per second.

   2. Muscle tremor (M.T.)—irregular jerks.

   3. Wandering baseline (W.B.).

5. Identify the artifacts in these tracings
   (A.C., M.T., W.B. or a combination).

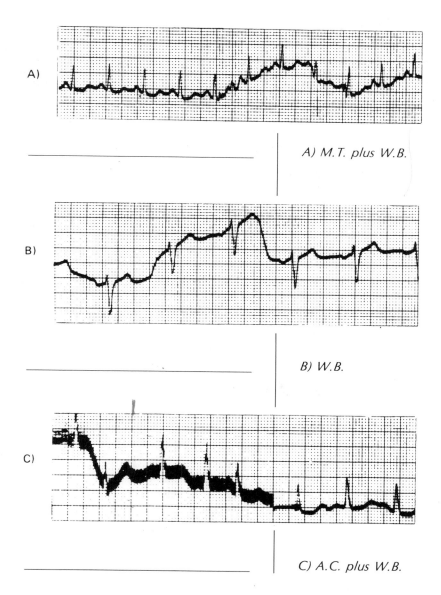

A)

B)

C)

A) M.T. plus W.B.

B) W.B.

C) A.C. plus W.B.

6.

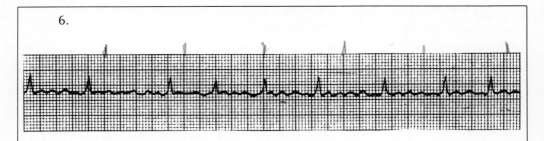

At this point in your training you may not be able to make a *diagnosis* of this arrhythmia, but you could give a *description* as follows:

Technique is satisfactory.

Ventricular rate is 85/min. There are 8.5 R-R intervals in 15 cm. (6 sec.). QRS duration is 0.08 sec.
QRS complexes are uniform in appearance. Ventricular rhythm is irregular. Since the rhythm is totally irregular, I can't really say that any one cycle is premature.
P waves are not seen. Atrial rhythm is uncertain, but there are small undulations of variable contour.

Given this *description* by telephone, the more experienced observer can be fairly certain the *diagnosis* is atrial fibrillation.

7.

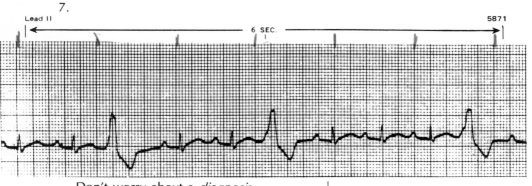

Lead II

6 SEC.

5871

Don't worry about a *diagnosis.*
Describe this monitoring lead as well as you can.

Technique	_____	*Satisfactory*
Ventricular rate	96 + /min.	*96/min.*
Ventricular rhythm	_____	*Rhythm basically regular, interrupted by three premature beats*
QRS duration	.04 sec.	*0.07 sec.*
Premature QRS complexes	_____	*Three premature QRS*
Do all QRS complexes have the same configuration?	prems .20 broad _____	*The premature complexes are broad (0.15 sec.) and "different."*
Atrial rate	_____ /min.	*96/min.*
Atrial rhythm	_____	*Probably regular; (P may be hidden in the premature complexes.)*
Any premature P waves?	_____	*No*
PR interval	.24 sec.	*0.23*
Conclusion	_____	*Regular rhythm is interrupted by three premature QRS complexes which are broad and different. They are not preceded by premature P waves. PR is longer than normal.*

8.

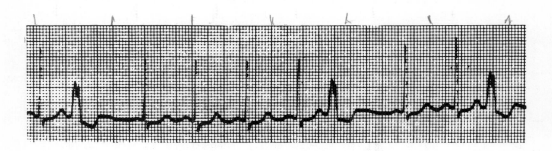

Describe this monitoring lead ECG as well as you can. (Write your own description before proceeding to the next page.)

Technique ____Satisfactory_____

QRS Complexes
Ventricular rate __105__ /min.   QRS duration __0.04__ /sec.
Ventricular rhythm _Reg. exc. for 3 prem Q's._

Premature QRS complexes _3 broad .16 sec double_
peaked No P waves.
Do all complexes have the same configuration? _Some taller than others._

Atrial Complexes
Atrial rate _105_ /min.
Atrial rhythm _reg._
Premature complexes _No._

A-V Conduction
PR interval _0.16_ sec. ☑ normal ☐ long ☐ short
                        ☑ constant   ☐ variable

Is each P wave followed by a QRS complex? _yes._

CONCLUSION _Three irreg QRS complex, prem._
broad, double peaked 5 preceding P waves

9.

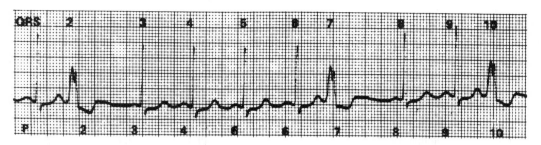

Technique—A little wandering baseline, but perfectly adequate for interpretation.

QRS Complexes

Ventricular rate—*94/min.*   QRS duration—*0.06 sec. for the dominant cycles, about 0.13 sec. for the premature cycles.*

Ventricular rhythm—*Fundamentally regular, but see below.*

Premature QRS complexes—*The 2nd, 7th and 10th are premature, broad and "different." They are not preceded by a premature P and they do not interrupt the atrial rhythm.*

Do all complexes have the same configuration?—*No. The premature complexes are "different."*

Atrial Complexes

Atrial rate—*94/min. P waves could be hidden in cycles 2, 7, and 10.*
Atrial rhythm—*Regular. The premature cycles do not interrupt the atrial rhythm.*
Premature P waves—*None.*

A-V Conduction

PR interval—*0.14 sec.*   [X] normal   [ ] long   [ ] short
                          [X] constant   [ ] variable

Is each P wave followed by a QRS complex?—*Yes, except for those which occur during the premature cycles.*

CONCLUSION—*Sinus rhythm. Rate 94/min. PR 0.14 sec. QRS 0.06 sec. The atrial rhythm is regular, but the 2nd, 7th, and 10th P waves are hidden in the premature and broad QRS complexes. These three P waves are not conducted. Three QRS complexes are premature, broad, "different" and are not preceded by premature P waves. They do not interrupt the atrial rhythm.*

SUMMARY—CHAPTER V

Regular use of this system for evaluating rhythm strips will help to avoid overlooking important features:

1. Is technique adequate for interpretation?

2. Determine ventricular rate, rhythm, and QRS duration.

3. Determine atrial rate and rhythm.

4. Evaluate atrio-ventricular relationship.

PROBLEMS—CHAPTER V

1. A 52-year-old man was about to be transferred from the Intensive Coronary Care area following myocardial infarction. The alarm sounded. This was the monitor record. Complete as much as you can of the ECG Description.

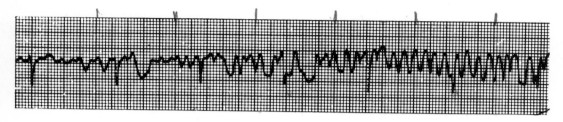

ECG DESCRIPTION

Technique _____ Satisfactory _____

QRS Complexes
Ventricular rate ___ 65 ___ /min.   QRS duration ___ 0.08 ___ /sec.
Ventricular rhythm ___ reg ___
Premature QRS complexes ___ no. ___
Do all complexes have the same configuration? ___ no. 4ᵗʰ 6ᵗʰ ___
broad + diff (double peaked)
dur = 0.16

Atrial Complexes
Atrial rate _____ /min.
Atrial rhythm _____
Premature beats _____

A-V Conduction
PR interval _____ sec.   ☐ normal   ☐ long   ☐ short
                             ☐ constant ☐ variable
Is each P wave followed by a QRS complex? _____

CONCLUSION _____
_____
_____

2. In approaching a rhythm strip systematically, the first step is to evaluate ___*tech*___ .

3. Ventricular complexes are studied next. Reasons for studying QRS before P include the following:

		True	False
A.	QRS is larger than P.	X	___
B.	QRS can be located in a hurry, even by a novice.	X	___
C.	The pumping function of the heart has a direct relationship to ventricular rate.	X	___
D.	Ventricular arrhythmias are of more immediate life-threatening importance than supraventricular arrhythmias.	X	___

chapter 6

sinus rhythms

1.

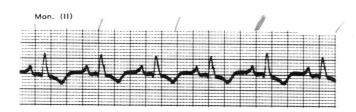

Mon. (II)

Normal sinus rhythm (NSR) is characterized by:

1. Upright P in a monitoring lead with lead II axis (right shoulder negative, left axilla positive). In lead MCL-1, sinus P waves may be negative or positive.

2. P-P interval fairly regular (plus or minus 10%).

3. P waves are uniform.

4. Each P is followed by a QRS and the PR interval is normal (0.12–0.20 sec.).

5. Rate between 60 and 100 per minute.

2. **Sinus rhythm** means that the sinus node is in control; it is the pacemaker.

The sinus node is at the head end of the atria.

Thus, an atrial depolarization wave starting in the sinus node will spread in a direction which is from

_____ foot to head.

___✓___ head to foot.   *head to foot.*

3. A commonly used monitoring lead has an axis similar to that of lead II.

In a monitoring lead with lead II axis, a P wave of sinus origin is

_____ negative.

___✓___ positive.   *positive.*

4.

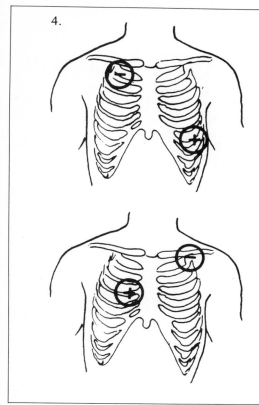

Mon (II)

This is the hook-up for a monitoring lead with an axis similar to that of lead II. In Mon. (II), a sinus P wave is positive.

MCL-1

This is the hook-up for an MCL-1 monitoring lead. The negative electrode is at the left shoulder. The positive electrode is in the fourth interspace at the right sternal border. The MCL-1 lead is most helpful for understanding certain problems of QRS configuration. In MCL-1, a sinus P wave may be positive or negative.

5.

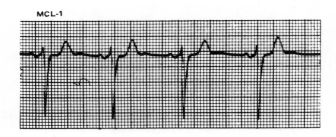

MCL-1

Note that this is lead MCL-1.

This could be sinus rhythm.

_____ ✓ _____ true.

_____ false.   *true.*

Why? _reg rhythm, P waves_

rate 60+ _precede QRS, neg (because MCL-1)_

PR interval 0.16 sec.

*P wave is diphasic in
this lead but it might
be upright in the lead II
axis.*

---

6. Tachycardia means fast rate—more than 100 per minute.

   Bradycardia means slow rate—less than 60 per minute.

---

7. An abnormally fast rhythm arising in the
   sinus node is called _tachyca_ .   *sinus tachycardia.*

8.

Mon. (II)

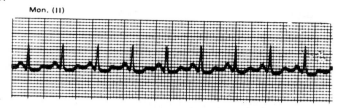

Sinus tachycardia is characterized by:

rate > 100/min,

reg. rhythm, p waves

followed by QRS

PR interval .12

Upright P in lead II.

P-P interval is fairly regular.

Each P is followed by a
QRS.

PR interval normal.

Rate over 100/min.

Mon. (II)   10-041-35

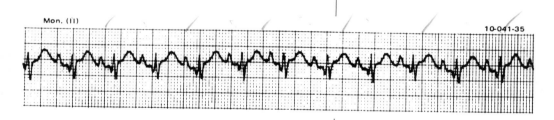

Does this meet the criteria of sinus tachycardia?

yes? (P-R interval short
?

Yes

9. What criteria would you expect for sinus
bradycardia?

reg rhythm, Normal P-P interval

normal P-R interval,
(lead II)

upright P followed by QRS,

rate < 60/min.

Upright P in lead II.
P-P interval is fairly
regular.
Each P is followed by a
QRS.
PR interval normal.
Rate below 60/min.

10.

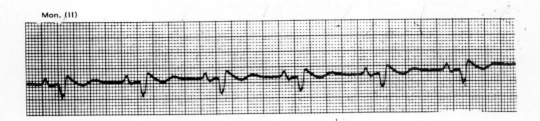

Does this meet the criteria of sinus brady-cardia?

rate over 60,

___NO___ | Yes

---

11. Though the fundamental atrial mechanism may be sinus rhythm, various arrhythmias may **interrupt** (such as premature complexes) or **coexist** (such as A-V block).

Sinus rhythm with premature QRS complexes.

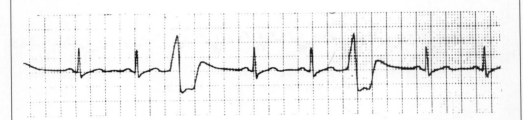

Atrial mechanism is sinus tachycardia but no P waves are conducted. Complete A-V block.

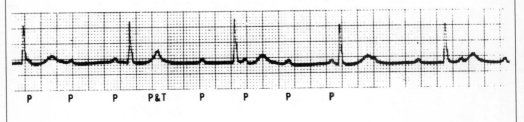

P   P   P   P&T   P   P   P   P

12. **Sinus rhythms usually are not precisely regular.** Often this helps to distinguish sinus tachycardia from tachycardia arising in an ectopic supraventricular focus (supraventricular tachycardia).

13.

Mon. (II)

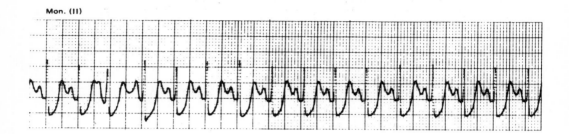

This rhythm strip shows several features of sinus tachycardia: (1) Rate above 100 (150/min.); (2) P waves upright and uniform; (3) _P-P interval fairly reg._

(3) Rhythm is not precisely regular.

14. **Sinus arrhythmia** is a sinus rhythm in which the P-P interval varies, usually at least 10%. Commonly the speeding and slowing are phasic, related to respiration.

Sinus arrhythmia is common in healthy people.

15. The only abnormality of sinus arrhythmia is

_____ inverted P waves.

___✓___ slight variation in P-P interval.

_____ broad QRS configuration.

slight variation in P-P interval.

16.

Mon. (II)

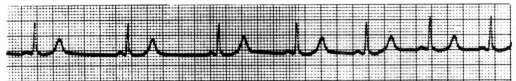

Sinus arrhythmia shows slight irregularity of the P-P interval. The P wave configuration

_____ varies from cycle to cycle.

___✓___ remains constant.

remains constant.

---

17. **Sinus pause** (or sinus arrest) describes the cessation of sinus node activity and thus the temporary disappearance of usual P waves.

This is uncommon in normal adults.

18.

Mon. (II)

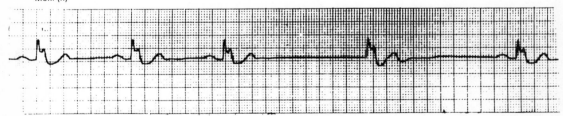

Regularly occurring sinus P waves suddenly stop, then resume in the latter part of this rhythm strip.

This indicates sinus _sinus pause_.

arrest (or sinus pause).

SUMMARY—CHAPTER VI

1. Sinus rhythm is fairly regular, not precisely regular. P waves are upright in lead II. Each P is followed by a QRS at a rate of 60–100/min.

2. Slight irregularity, usually phasic with respiration, is expected with sinus rhythms. When marked, the respiratory variation is termed sinus arrhythmia.

3. The sinus node does not produce premature cycles, but it may pause, arrest, or cause bradycardia or tachycardia.

PROBLEMS—CHAPTER VI

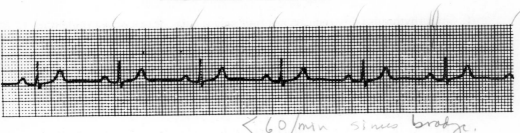

< 60/min sinus brady.

1. Conclusion: _normal sinus rhythms_

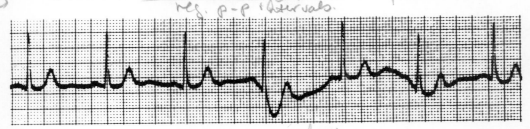

164-268

a   b   c   d   e   f   g   h   i

hidden p   hidden p   hidden p

(sinus pause?)

prem QRS - count a part - rate?

2. Conclusion: _Sinus brad arrthm   ī prem. QRS_
reg. p-p intervals.

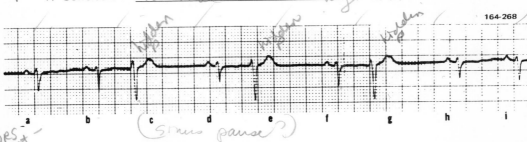

3. Conclusion: _normal sinus rhythm_   artifact (wandering base)

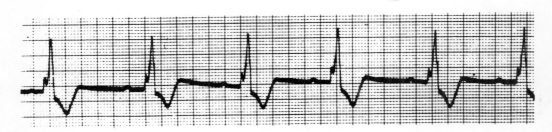

4. Conclusion: _sinus bradycardia_
Long P-R interval
& wide QRS

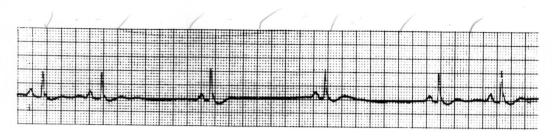

5. Conclusion: _____sinus bradya_____ sinus arrhyth

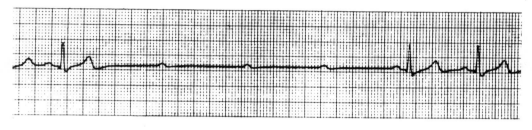

6. Conclusion: _____AV block._____

chapter 7

an introduction to arrhythmias

A review of normal rhythmicity will help to understand the abnormal.

> 1. Under normal circumstances, if a faster or slower heart rate is required, this is provided by chemical and nerve reflex action on the sinus node. The rate of discharge of the sinus node normally controls the heart.

2. If your heart rate speeds to 122/min. after exercise, the cause probably is

_____ activity of an ectopic focus.

_____ acceleration of sinus node discharge rate through chemical and reflex changes brought about by exertion.

acceleration of sinus node.

DORMANT PACEMAKERS

3. Although the sinus node usually is in charge, other foci are ready, willing, and anxious to take over! Other pacing foci exist in the atria, the junctional tissue, and the ventricles. These are spoken of as **ectopic foci** because they are outside the normal pacemaker location in the sinus node. They remain dormant because they regularly are discharged by the sinus impulse. The natural rate of discharge of these lower pacemaking centers is slower than the natural rate of discharge of the sinus node.

The **inherent discharge rate** of a pacing focus describes its natural **automaticity.**

Imagine a long-dormant pacing center in the junctional tissue, just waiting for a chance to produce a heartbeat of its own. Slowly it builds up a charge, getting ready to release an impulse. However, as usual, the sinus node builds up its charge first, releases it and depolarizes the lower center before it has a chance to become manifest. Then the process starts all over again, for the sinus node has greater automaticity than the A-V junction.

4. What do you expect might happen if the sinus node fails to discharge or if the sinus impulse is blocked some place along its way to the lower regions?

_____

_____

One of the lower centers might have a chance to release its impulse and control the heart cycle.

5. Mechanisms which cause arrhythmias include:

   1. Default or slowing of the sinus node.

   2. Failure of conduction of the sinus impulse.

   3. Escape of a lower focus.

   4. Enhanced automaticity of an ectopic focus.

   5. Reentry.

6. Imagine that the sinus node becomes sick, damaged or poisoned. Now some lower focus has a chance.

   Escape is the term used to describe an ectopic rhythm which develops through default of a higher focus or through failure of conduction (block) of the normal impulse from above.

7. The organization of the special cardiac tissues provides that the lower the focus, the slower the automatic rate.

8. DISCHARGE RATE

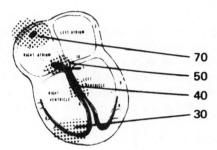

70
50
40
30

If the normal sinus rate is about 70, an escape focus in the junctional tissue might have a rate of 40 to 60, in the bundle of His perhaps 30 to 40, and low in the ventricles perhaps _____ /min.

20 or 30/min.

9. Thus far we have discussed three mechanisms which might be responsible for arrhythmias.

   1. _____

   2. _____

   3. _____

1. failure of sinus node to discharge.

2. block of a normal sinus impulse.

3. escape of a lower focus through default or block above.

10. Another cause of arrhythmias is an abnormally fast discharge rate of an ectopic focus. This is called **enhanced automaticity.**

    Disease or drugs may cause enhanced automaticity of a lower center. A single premature complex or a bout of tachycardia may result.

11.

Sinus cycles.   **A burst of tachycardia.**

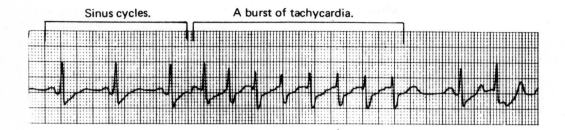

Sinus rhythm is interrupted by a burst of tachycardia. This arrhythmia might be due to

_____ enhanced automaticity.

_____ escape.

enhanced automaticity. (Note that the first complex of the paroxysm occurs prematurely. This is a sign of enhanced activity of an arrhythmic focus.)

12.

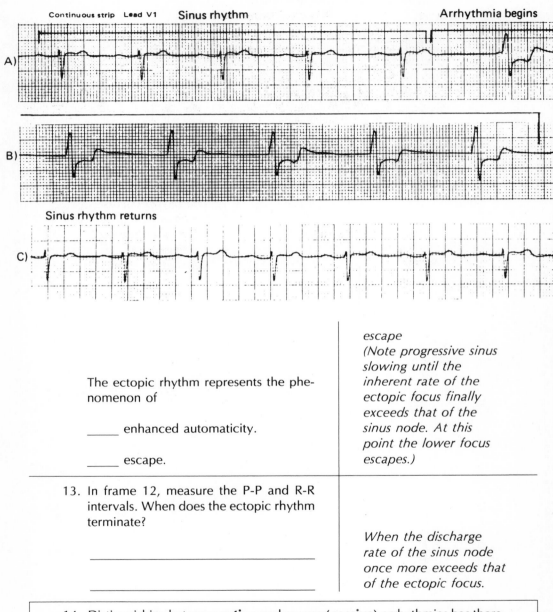

Continuous strip   Lead V1   **Sinus rhythm**   **Arrhythmia begins**

A)

B)

Sinus rhythm returns

C)

The ectopic rhythm represents the phenomenon of

_____ enhanced automaticity.

_____ escape.

escape
(Note progressive sinus
slowing until the
inherent rate of the
ectopic focus finally
exceeds that of the
sinus node. At this
point the lower focus
escapes.)

13. In frame 12, measure the P-P and R-R intervals. When does the ectopic rhythm terminate?

_____

_____

When the discharge
rate of the sinus node
once more exceeds that
of the ectopic focus.

14. Distinguishing between **active** and escape **(passive)** arrhythmias has therapeutic importance, especially in the CCU. Enhanced automaticity causing an active arrhythmia requires a depressant drug. An arrhythmia due to escape is best handled by speeding the heart rate.

15. If the arrhythmia shown in frame 12 needs treatment, a logical choice might be

_____ a drug to **speed** the sinus rate (atropine).

_____ a drug to **suppress** an ectopic focus (lidocaine).

atropine.

16.

10-28-27

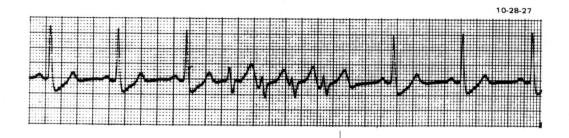

This arrhythmia might be treated wisely with

_____ an accelerator of the sinus node.

_____ a suppressant of ectopic foci.

a suppressant of ectopic foci.

REENTRY

17. Reentry is another mechanism of arrhythmias. It may cause a premature complex or a bout of tachycardia. The sketch may help to visualize one concept of reentrant arrhythmias.

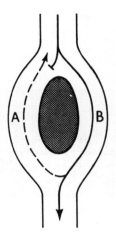

Suppose a downcoming impulse from the atria reaches a division in the conducting pathways in the A-V junction. Suppose path A blocks forward (antegrade) conduction but permits retrograde conduction. Part of the depolarization wave might reenter the atria, causing a premature atrial complex. If the process were repeated, a bout of atrial tachycardia might result.

18.

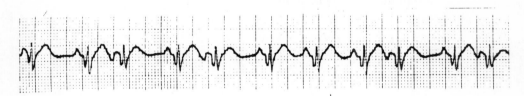

The premature complexes in this strip might be due to

_____ enhanced automaticity.

_____ reentry.

Either mechanism is possible.

TYPES OF ARRHYTHMIAS

19. It is reassuring to know that the great majority of arrhythmias with which we will deal on an everyday basis are quite straightforward.

    The **types of straightforward arrhythmias** include: tachycardia, brady-cardia, premature complexes, flutter, fibrillation, conduction disorders, and standstill.

20. Since arrhythmias arise from a limited number of sites, the number of labels to deal with is not excessive.

    The **sites** from which arrhythmias may arise are: the sinus node, atria, A-V junction, or ventricles.

    Most arrhythmias are labeled as to site and type. **Mechanism** is a more common word than type in this connection.

21. Sinus tachycardia is a common arr-hythmia.

    In this label, which word refers to *site?*

    _____

    Which word refers to *mechanism* of ar-rhythmia?   _____

    sinus

    tachycardia

22. Examples of arrhythmias according to site of origin and mechanism include the following:

SITE	MECHANISM
Sinus	tachycardia
Sinus	bradycardia
Sinus	arrest
Sinus	arrhythmia
Atrial	premature complex
Atrial*	tachycardia
Atrial	flutter
Atrial	fibrillation
A-V junctional**	tachycardia
A-V junctional	premature beat
A-V	block
Ventricular	premature complex
Ventricular	tachycardia
Ventricular	flutter
Ventricular	fibrillation
Ventricular	standstill (arrest)

*Supraventricular tachycardia is the term preferred by some.

**We use the following terms interchangeably: junctional, A-V nodal, A-V junctional.

23. Some *key questions.*

It is helpful to **classify an arrhythmia** by asking some key questions.

1. What is the site and mechanism?

2. Is it supraventricular or ventricular?

3. Is it passive (due to escape), or is it active (due to enhanced automaticity)?

4. Is impaired conduction the problem?

24.

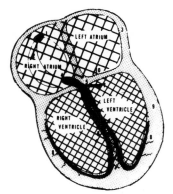

A **supraventricular arrhythmia** is one which originates in the sinus node, atria or A-V junctional apparatus.

A **ventricular arrhythmia** originates in the ventricles.

Distinction between supraventricular and ventricular arrhythmias has much therapeutic importance. The distinction often can be made on the basis of QRS duration.

25. Think of site and mechanism. List three supraventricular arrhythmias.

_____

_____

_____

SITE	MECHANISM
sinus	tachycardia
sinus	bradycardia
atrial	tachycardia
atrial	premature complex
atrial	fibrillation
junctional	tachycardia
junctional	premature complex

26. In determining therapy, it is important to know whether the arrhythmia is ventricular or supraventricular. Often this can be determined simply on the basis of duration of the _____.

QRS complex

27. Spread of the depolarization wave through the ventricles causes a QRS complex. If spread is rapid, QRS is narrow—0.10 sec. or less. If spread is slow, QRS is broad—0.11 sec. or more.

28. Normally the depolarization wave gets through the ventricles in _____ sec. or less.

0.10

29. Generally speaking, the only way a depolarization wave can get through the ventricles rapidly (in 0.10 sec. or less) is to utilize the rapidly conducting His-Purkinje system. To utilize the His-Purkinje system fully, the depolarization wave must come down from above. Only impulses of supraventricular origin can utilize the His-Purkinje system.

30. Supraventricular rhythms are sinus, atrial, or junctional.

31. If QRS is narrow, the impulse causing it must have started in the junctional apparatus, atria, or _____.

sinus node.

32. What about a broad QRS? A broad QRS indicates slow distribution of the depolarization wave.

There are two possibilities.

1. The impulse arose in the ventricle itself and was distributed throughout the ventricles via the slowly conducting, ordinary muscle fibers.

2. Or, perhaps a supraventricular impulse, descending from above, finds part of the His-Purkinje system partly or completely blocked. The affected portion of the ventricles must be supplied via the slowly conducting ordinary muscle fibers. Traveling a round-about route over slow roads, the impulse has a long traveling time.

33. Thus, to approach an arrhythmia, study the QRS complex.

    A **narrow QRS** is of supraventricular origin.
    The rapidly conducting His-Purkinje system can be utilized only if the excitation wave comes down from above.

    A **broad QRS** has two possible origins. It could be

    ventricular
    or
    supraventricular with abnormal (aberrant) ventricular conduction.

34. A narrow QRS

    _____ always is of supraventricular origin.

    _____ could be of ventricular origin.

    always is of supraventricular origin. (It is dangerous to say **always.** *However, take that risk and assume that a narrow QRS means rapid spread via a normal His-Purkinje system, and this means supraventricular origin.)*

35. A broad QRS

    _____ always is of ventricular origin.

    _____ could be of supraventricular origin.

    could be of supraventricular origin if ventricular conduction is abnormal.

36.

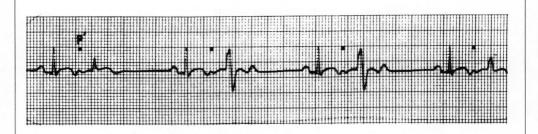

Ectopic ventricular complexes are broad and bizarre. However, not all broad and bizarre QRS complexes are of ectopic ventricular origin. One must always consider supraventricular origin with aberrant (abnormal) ventricular conduction.

In this illustration, note the premature P responsible for each of the anomalous QRS complexes. Since QRS follows P we assume the premature QRS resulted from a premature atrial systole. QRS is broad because of aberrant conduction through the ventricles. This is the topic of the next chapter.

---

37. An early complex which arises in the atria is called an _____ premature complex.

atrial

38.

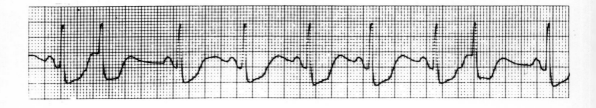

The two premature complexes

_____ must be of supraventricular origin.

_____ could be of ventricular origin.

must be of supraventricular origin (as they are narrow).

39. A rapid rhythm arising from an ectopic focus in the atrial muscle is

    _____ sinus tachycardia.

    _____ atrial tachycardia.   *atrial tachycardia.*

---

40. A tachycardia which comes and goes in brief episodes is paroxysmal. A paroxysmal tachycardia

    _____ starts suddenly.

    _____ lasts minutes or hours.   *starts suddenly.*

    _____ comes in episodes.   *lasts minutes or hours.*

    _____ has a rate of 100 or less.   *comes in episodes.*

SUPRAVENTRICULAR TACHYCARDIA

41. An ectopic tachycardia arising above the ventricles is called a supraventricular tachycardia. Either atrial muscle or A-V node may be responsible.

    The term supraventricular tachycardia is used when a more specific diagnosis is not possible.

---

42. A supraventricular tachycardia may arise in the

    _____ atria.

    _____ ventricle.   *atria.*

    _____ A-V junction.   *A-V junction.*

---

43. Many tachycardias arise from repeated discharge of a single focus.

    Sinus tachycardia arises from the sinus node. All other tachycardias arise from an abnormal or ectopic focus.

44. A single focus with increased automaticity may cause

   _____ a single ectopic impulse.

   _____ a short series of ectopic impulses.

   _____ a long run of tachycardia.

   All three choices are correct.

45. The reentry phenomenon could cause

   _____ a single ectopic impulse.

   _____ a short series of ectopic impulses.

   _____ a long run of tachycardia.

   All three choices are correct.

LADDER DIAGRAM

46.

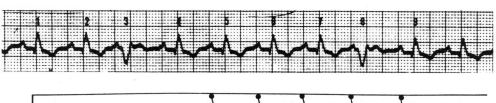

First, draw only what you can see. Start with QRS. In the rung marked "ventricle," make a slash corresponding to each QRS. If QRS is **narrow,** undoubtedly it is of supraventricular origin and the slash runs downward. If QRS is **broad,** final decision may have to wait, but in this instance, QRS No. 3 has all the earmarks of ectopic ventricular origin. Thus the slash is shown running upward. (QRS entries have been made for cycles 2—4.)

Second, indicate each P wave with a slash in the atrial rung. It runs downward unless you suspect retrograde spread from a ventricular or junctional origin. (P wave entries have been made for cycles 5 and 6.)

Finally, connect the atrial and ventricular slashes as seems appropriate. Events in the A-V junction can only be inferred. Thus, they are left to last. (A full ladder has been drawn for cycles 7 and 9.)

SUMMARY—CHAPTER VII

1. Failure of sinus discharge or of conduction may permit escape of a lower, dormant pacemaker.

2. Enhanced automaticity of an ectopic focus or the reentry phenomenon account for premature complexes or ectopic tachycardia.

3. Rhythm diagnoses usually indicate site and mechanism, e.g., atrial flutter.

4. Because atrial and junctional rhythms often cannot be distinguished, the vague and inclusive term supraventricular is useful.

5. If QRS is narrow, the arrhythmia is **supraventricular.** If QRS is broad and "different," the arrhythmia is either **ventricular** OR **supraventricular with abnormal ventricular conduction.**

PROBLEMS—CHAPTER VII

1. A rhythm initiated by the sinus node is called sinus rhythm. A rhythm initiated elsewhere in the heart is called an _____ rhythm. Rhythms may arise in the atrial muscle, the A-V junction, or the ventricles.

2. Potential pacing foci in atria, junctional tissue, and ventricles normally are dormant because they regularly are discharged by impulses initiated in the _____ . If the sinus node does not discharge fast enough, a lower focus may escape.

3. At different levels of the heart, the natural rate of automatic discharge varies. The natural rate of the sinus node is about 50–100/min. A junctional escape focus will have a rate of 40–60/min. and a ventricular escape focus is likely to have a rate of _____ /min.

4. Enhanced _____ is the problem when an ectopic focus is responsible for a premature impulse or a bout of tachycardia. Reentry also can cause premature complexes or tachycardia.

5. Mechanisms responsible for arrhythmias include:

   1. Sinus arrest or failure of conduction of a normal impulse.
   2. Escape of a lower focus, an example of a passive arrhythmia.
   3. Enhanced _____ , the phenomenon responsible for some active arrhythmias.
   4. The reentry phenomenon.

6. Determining whether an arrhythmia arises in supraventricular or ventricular tissues often is of major therapeutic importance. Usually this can be done by determining whether QRS is _____ or _____ .

7.

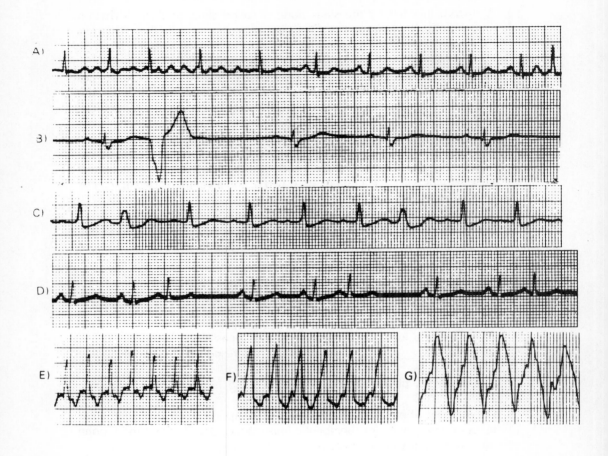

Which of the above arrhythmias can only be supraventricular? _____.

Which could be either ventricular or supraventricular with abnormal ventricular conduction? _____ .

8.

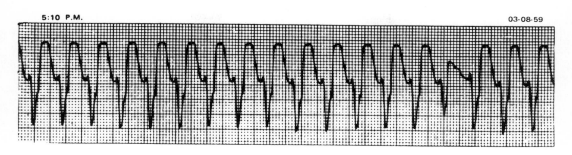

QRS duration appears to be about 0.11 sec. Elsewhere in a 12-lead tracing, QRS duration clearly was 0.13 sec. No P waves are seen. Even if P waves are present we seldom expect to find them when the rate is this rapid.

From what has been presented so far, could the focus for this tachycardia be in the ventricles? _____

Could the focus be supraventricular? _____

chapter 8

bundle branch block and aberrant ventricular conduction

1. The right and left bundle branches (RBB and LBB) are part of the His-Purkinje system. This **specialized conduction apparatus** permits rapid ventricular distribution of an impulse of supraventricular origin.

2. When the freeway is blocked, you will need extra time to get home. A detour prolongs your trip for two reasons:

   1. _____

   2. _____

   1. A roundabout path requires extra mileage.

   2. Back roads are slow.

3. If a portion of the bundle branch system is blocked, excitation of the affected part of the ventricle is delayed. The depolarization wave must detour, spread through ordinary, slowly conducting muscle fibers. As a result, when a supraventricular impulse encounters block in one of the bundle branches, the QRS complex is prolonged.

4. QRS is broadened in BBB because the depolarization wave must utilize:

 1. a roundabout route.

 2. ordinary muscle fibers. These conduct

 _____ slower than

 _____ faster than

 the His-Purkinje fibers.

 | *slower than* |

---

5. In right bundle branch block (RBBB), depolarization is delayed in the

 _____ right

 _____ left

 ventricle.

 | *right* |

---

6. In BBB, the affected ventricle is finally activated when the depolarization wave reaches it via the uninvolved ventricle. This process requires a longer time than normal and results in a QRS which is

 _____ longer in duration.

 _____ shorter in duration.

 | *longer in duration.* |

---

7. When ventricular depolarization is slow, the QRS complex is likely to be

 _____ 0.06 sec.

 _____ 0.08 sec.

 _____ 0.13 sec.

 | *0.13 sec.* |

---

8. In BBB, a ventricle is depolarized via a different route. Thus, the QRS configuration is broad and _____.

 | *"different."* |

9. QRS configuration is "different" in BBB because

_____ depolarization pathways are "different."

_____ infarction probably caused the block.

depolarization pathways are "different."

10. Our chief interest in BBB is the confusion it causes in dealing with a broad QRS tachycardia. "Is it ventricular tachycardia or supraventricular tachycardia with BBB?"

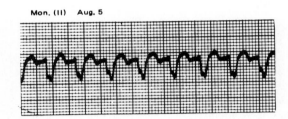

Mon. (II)   Aug. 5

There are two possibilities:

1. The impulse arose in the ventricles and thus was distributed via slowly conducting ordinary muscle fibers; or

2. The impulse arose in a supraventricular focus but encountered block in one of the bundles.

11.

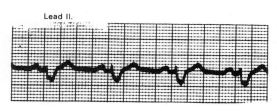

Lead II.

This is from the same patient shown in frame 10. Sinus rhythm is present. The broad QRS indicates _____.

BBB.

The tachycardia of Aug. 5 must have been

_____ supraventricular with BBB.

_____ ventricular.

supraventricular with BBB.

12. Conduction may be blocked completely or just delayed.

An entire bundle may be involved or just one of its divisions (fascicles). Related terms include **fascicular block, divisional block, hemiblock,** incomplete block.

Although delay in one small fascicle does not produce obvious QRS widening, the altered sequence of ventricular activation may produce marked change in QRS configuration.

13. This man was admitted July 2 with acute infarction. Note the marked QRS changes as conduction abnormalities (fascicular block) varied from day to day. These changes are due to altered sequence of ventricular activation from one day to the next. On July 2, there was late activation of the **inferior** portion of the left ventricular (inferior hemiblock); on July 3 there was late activation of the **superior** portion of the left ventricle.

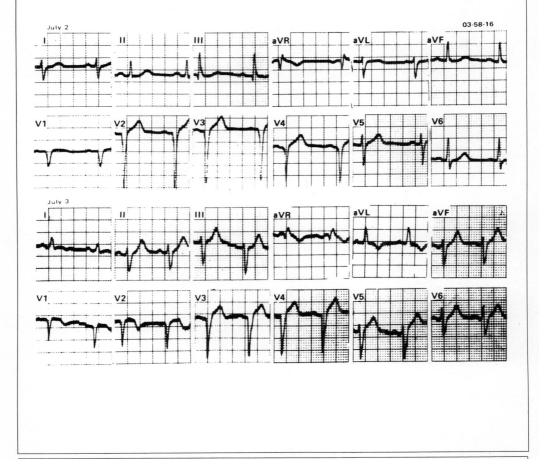

14. QRS represents depolarization; **ST-T represents repolarization.** When **de**polarization pathways change, **re**polarization pathways also change.

15.

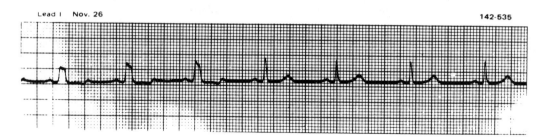

Lead I   Nov. 26   142-535

In this patient, BBB is intermittent.

As QRS changes, note the change in ST-T.

ST-T features are altered by BBB because

_____ ischemia ordinarily accompanies conduction abnormality.

_____ altered depolarization is followed by altered repolarization.

altered depolarization is followed by altered repolarization.

16. A QRS of "different" configuration often is described as **"anomalous."**

Impaired conduction need not be due to anatomic or mechanical interruption of a bundle; it may be functional rather than organic.

This introduces a new term, **refractory period.**

17. After the conduction apparatus is depolarized, it is totally unable to conduct again for a brief period. This is called the **absolute refractory period.**

After a little more recuperation, it is able to conduct but does so slowly. This is the **relative refractory period.**

Different divisions of the conduction system have different rest requirements. One division may be fully recovered and able to conduct normally. Other sections may conduct slowly or not at all.

18. **Aberrant ventricular conduction** (AVC) describes the "different" QRS configuration which occurs when a portion of the His-Purkinje system is partially refractory at the time of arrival of a supraventricular impulse. For one or for a series of cycles, QRS morphology is that of BBB or incomplete BBB.

    Because the right bundle commonly has the longer refractory period (rest requirement), AVC most often resembles right BBB.

AVC VS. BBB

19. Aberrant ventricular conduction (AVC) is related to bundle branch block.

    In common usage, BBB describes the situation in which a bundle fails to conduct even though rest time since the prior impulse should have been adequate for full recovery. BBB usually is **permanent.**

    Aberrant ventricular conduction is **temporary,** often present for a single complex. AVC describes poor conduction due to early arrival of the supraventricular impulse, while part of the bundle is still refractory. Because the right bundle has a longer refractory period (rest requirement) than the left, AVC most often is due to delayed activation of the right ventricle.

20. When a bundle conducts poorly because a supraventricular impulse came down too soon after the preceding cycle, aberrant ventricular conduction results. Rest time was inadequate and a portion of the bundle was still _____.   *refractory.*

21. The right bundle system has a longer rest requirement (a longer refractory period) than the left.

    Thus aberrant conduction usually is due to delay in the right bundle.

    AVC usually causes QRS features similar to those found in right BBB.

22. In RBBB or AVC, due to delay in the right bundle system, the right ventricle is depolarized last. The last part of QRS then represents right ventricular activation.

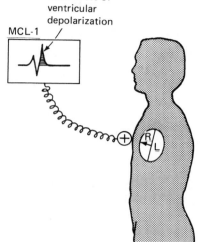

Last forces of ventricular depolarization

MCL-1

The right ventricle is an anterior chamber. Thus the last forces of ventricular activation are spreading anteriorly.

In leads MCL-1 and V1, the positive electrode is directly over the right ventricle.

In MCL-1, the last part of QRS is positive when AVC or BBB is due to delay in the right bundle system.

23. A depolarization wave spreading toward a positive electrode produces a

_____ positive

_____ negative   *positive*

deflection.

24. An advantage of the MCL-1 monitoring lead is that in this system the positive electrode is in the V1 position, directly over the right ventricle.

25. When AVC is due to delay in the right bundle system, in V1 or MCL-1, the last part of QRS will be

_____ positive.

_____ negative.   *positive.*

26.

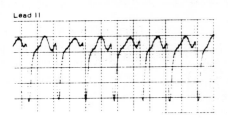

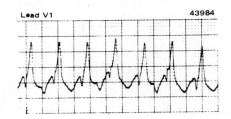

The above strip is particularly suggestive of supraventricular tachycardia with AVC because _____ .

the last part of QRS is positive in lead V1.

---

27. Recall that a positive deflection in a QRS complex is called an R wave. If there are two positive waves, the second is called "R-prime" (written R').

---

28. The QRS in lead V1 in frame 26 could be described as

_____ QR.

_____ RSR'.

_____ RS.

RSR'.

29. Although a broad, bizarre or "different" QRS usually is of ectopic ventricular origin, always consider supraventricular origin with aberrant ventricular conduction.

If you are considering supraventricular origin, ask two questions:

1. "Is the anomalous QRS preceded by a premature P wave?" The lead II axis may provide the best answer for this question.

2. "Does the anomalous QRS show late activation of the right ventricle?" Lead MCL-1 will provide the best answer to this question.

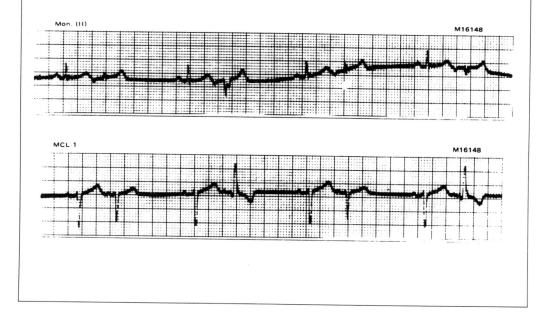

Mon. (II)   M16148

MCL-1   M16148

SUMMARY—CHAPTER VIII

1. A QRS of supraventricular origin is narrow. All narrow QRS complexes are of supraventricular origin.

2. A QRS of ventricular origin is broad. However, **broadness also may be due to aberrant ventricular conduction of a supraventricular impulse.**

3. Aberrant ventricular conduction should be considered in the differential diagnosis of all tachycardias with broad QRS.

4. Aberrant ventricular conduction also must be considered in the differential diagnosis of premature complexes which are broad and different.

5. A QRS of "different" configuration often is described as anomalous.

6. The right bundle system has a longer refractory period than the left. This means that a premature impulse is more likely to find the right bundle system incompletely recovered. Hence a RBBB pattern is expected with AVC.

7. Since the right ventricle is anterior, delay in right ventricular activation will cause terminal QRS forces to be oriented anteriorly. This causes a terminal R in lead MCL-1 or V1.

8. Thus, when QRS is anomalous, an RSR' configuration in MCL-1 or V1 is a hint that AVC is a more likely cause than ventricular ectopy.

9. Bundle branch block describes a more or less permanent conduction defect of one bundle. The ventricle it should supply is activated in roundabout fashion. The resultant QRS is broad and different.

PROBLEMS—CHAPTER VIII

Lead I.

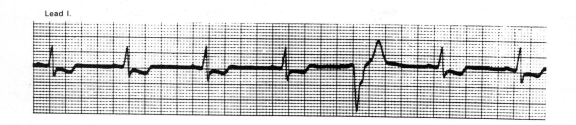

1. The QRS duration in the sinus cycles is 0.09 sec. Could this be BBB?

_____

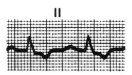 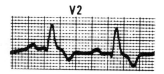

2. 1. What is the QRS duration?   _____ sec.

   2. Is bundle branch block present?   _____

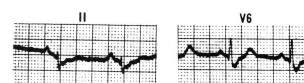

3. 1. What is the QRS duration?   _____ sec.

   2. Is bundle branch block present?   _____

Continuous strip

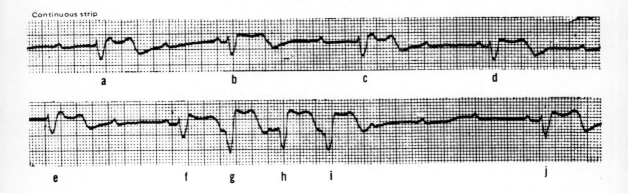

4. Does this show bundle branch block? _____

chapter 9

atrial and junctional premature complexes (supraventricular premature complexes)

1. The term **supraventricular arrhythmia** refers to those arrhythmias which arise any place above the first branching of the His bundle—in the atria, the A-V junction or in the common bundle itself.

   Supraventricular arrhythmias can utilize the His-Purkinje system. These are the arrhythmias with normal QRS duration.

2. If QRS is narrow, normal or the same as in the sinus complexes, the cycle

   _____ must be of supraventricular origin.

   _____ could be ventricular or supraventricular in origin.

   must be of supraventricular origin.

3. Normal QRS duration indicates supraventricular origin because only then can the His-Purkinje system be utilized normally for rapid ventricular activation.

4. An ectopic focus in the atria, junction, or ventricles may discharge prior to the expected discharge of the sinus node. If so, we will see ECG signs of an atrial, junctional, or ventricular premature complex.

The sinus node apparently does not release premature impulses.

5. Which of the following may give rise to supraventricular premature impulses?

_____ A-V junction

_____ bundle of His

_____ ventricles

_____ sinus node

_____ internodal and sino-atrial tracts

A-V junction

bundle of His

internodal and sino-atrial tracts

6. Atrial and junctional premature impulses activate the ventricles normally, via the His-Purkinje system. The QRS configuration is the same as in the sinus cycles (unless aberrant ventricular conduction occurs).

QRS is broad and "different" when the ventricles are activated via an abnormal route—due to an ectopic ventricular focus, BBB, or aberrant ventricular conduction.

7.

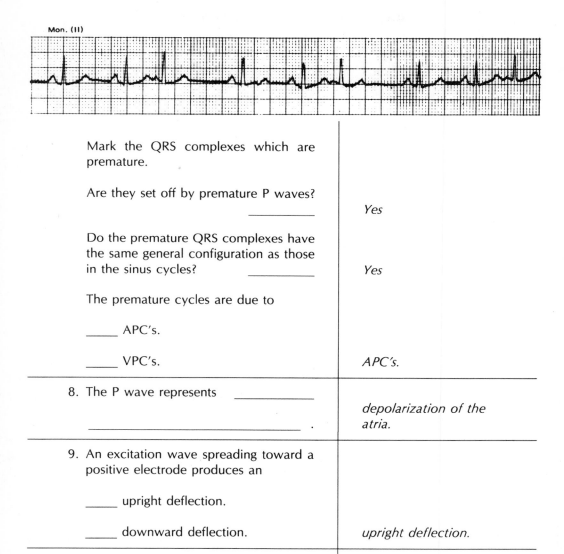

Mon. (II)

Mark the QRS complexes which are premature.

Are they set off by premature P waves?

_____   *Yes*

Do the premature QRS complexes have the same general configuration as those in the sinus cycles? _____   *Yes*

The premature cycles are due to

_____ APC's.

_____ VPC's.   *APC's.*

---

8. The P wave represents _____

_____ .   *depolarization of the atria.*

---

9. An excitation wave spreading toward a positive electrode produces an

_____ upright deflection.

_____ downward deflection.   *upright deflection.*

---

10. If atrial excitation starts in the head end of the atria, P wave direction in the monitoring lead with a lead II axis is

_____.   *upright.*

11. An atrial depolarization wave of ectopic origin may have a direction of spread similar to that of a sinus beat; if so, the P wave will be upright.

However, usually the direction of spread is altered and the P configuration in the APC is different from that of a sinus cycle.

---

12. Configuration of an ectopic P wave is likely to be

_____ identical to that of the sinus P wave.

_____ different from that of the sinus P wave.

different from that of the sinus P wave.

---

13. Simultaneous lead II (top) and lead V1 (below).

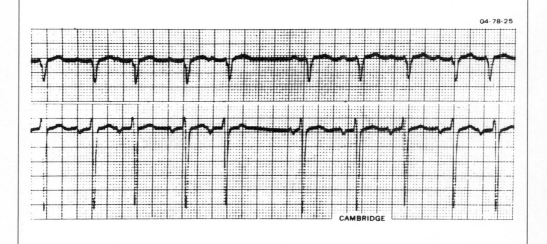

04-78-25

CAMBRIDGE

Both the sinus and the premature P waves are upright.

Whether or not premature P waves are inverted or otherwise "different" depends upon lead axis as well as the direction of atrial depolarization.

---

14. The PR interval represents _____

_____

_____ .

time required for spread of excitation through the atria, the A-V junction and His-Purkinje system.

15. The length of the PR interval associated with an APC is influenced by the site of the ectopic focus as well as the speed of conduction through the atria and A-V junction.

16. The PR interval of an APC could be

_____ longer than

_____ shorter than

_____ equal to

the PR interval of a normal sinus beat.

All three choices are correct.

17. The PR interval associated with an APC may be prolonged if the premature impulse finds the A-V junctional tissue incompletely recovered (partially refractory) following transmission of the prior impulse.

18.

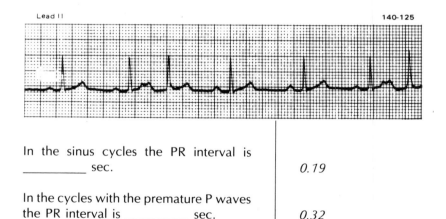

Lead II   140-125

In the sinus cycles the PR interval is
_____ sec.

0.79

In the cycles with the premature P waves
the PR interval is _____ sec.

0.32

BLOCKED APC'S

19. A premature P may occur so early in the refractory period of the junctional tissue that transmission to the ventricles is blocked.

When wondering about the **cause of a pause,** think of a **blocked APC.**

20.

Lead V1.

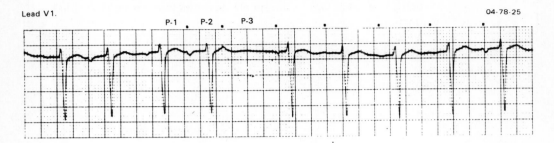

P-1   P-2   P-3   04-78-25

In this strip P-1 is of sinus origin.

The PR interval is _____   *0.16 sec*

P-2 is an APC. It comes so early it finds the A-V junction incompletely recovered.

The PR interval is _____   *0.26 sec.*

P-3 is an APC. It occurs so soon after the prior cycle that the conduction apparatus is totally refractory. The P is not conducted to the ventricles; it is blocked.

ESOPHAGEAL LEAD

21. Special leads may be needed to reveal the P waves.

   An electrode can be passed into the esophagus. The **esophageal lead** will demonstrate P waves of large amplitude because of proximity of the electrode to the left atrium.

   Simultaneous Mon. (II) (top) and esophageal lead (below).

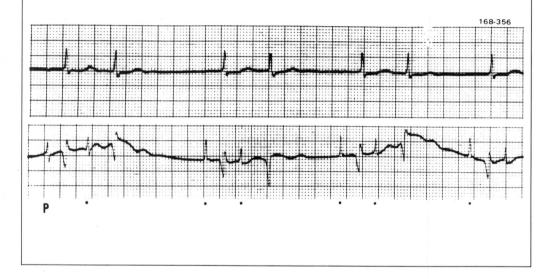

168-356

P

22. Simultaneous Mon. (II) (top) and esophageal lead (below).

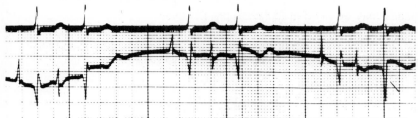

Premature P waves are not seen in Mon.
(II).

Label the P waves in the esophageal lead.

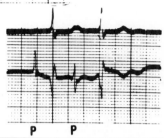

P   P

RIGHT ATRIAL ELECTROGRAM

23. Large P waves also are recorded from within the right atrium. Using a
transvenous pacing catheter as a recording electrode from the right atrium
often is more rapid and more comfortable than inserting the esophageal
electrode.

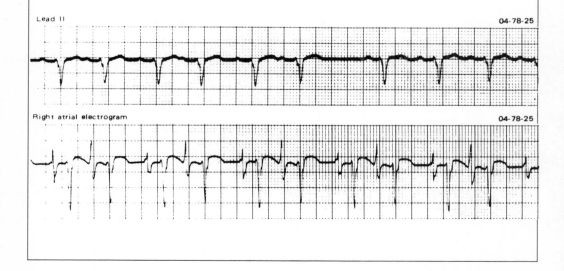

24.

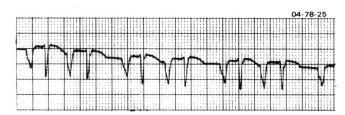

04-78-25

Label the P waves in this tracing recorded from an electrode catheter in the superior vena cava.

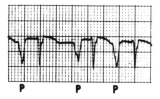

APC'S WITH ABERRANT VENTRICULAR CONDUCTION

25. Usually, the QRS complex due to an APC is identical to the QRS in the sinus cycles.

However, when a premature atrial impulse reaches the bundles or Purkinje fibers, these may still be recovering from recent transmission of the previous cycle. They may be "tired" (partially refractory). If the conduction tissue is **partially refractory,** conduction through the ventricles will be **aberrant.** The resultant QRS will be broader and "different" **(anomalous).**

26.

Lead VI

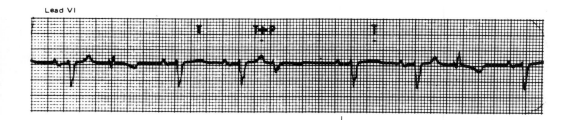

There are three APC's. Each of the premature QRS complexes is preceded by a premature P wave.

The premature complexes are anomalous due to _____ .

aberrant ventricular conduction.

ABERRANT CONDUCTION DUE TO BLOCK IN RIGHT BUNDLE

27. At least 8 times out of 10, AVC is associated with a **right** BBB pattern.

---

28. Aberrant ventricular conduction

_____ always

_____ usually

usually

causes a right bundle branch block pattern.

---

29. The right ventricle is anterior. If activation of the right ventricle is delayed, the last part of QRS in MCL-1 will be

_____ positive.

_____ negative.

positive.

30.

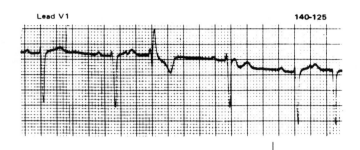

Lead V1   140-125

Complex No. 3 is premature, broad, "different," and preceded by a premature P. It is an APC with

_____ .

aberrant ventricular conduction.

The last forces of ventricular depolarization are directed toward the

_____ right ventricle.

_____ left ventricle.

right ventricle.

31. However, remember that **aberrant conduction does not always cause a right bundle branch block pattern** (RSR' in V1 or MCL-1).

32.

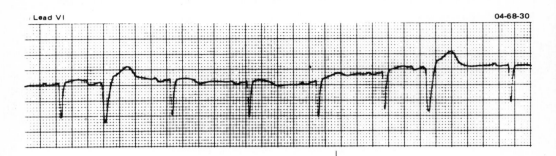

The premature QRS complexes are due to

_____ VPC's.

_____ APC's.

APC's with aberrant ventricular conduction, not of the RBBB variety.

PREMATURE P HIDDEN IN PRIOR T

33. We have learned one hint regarding APC's: the QRS may be anomalous, often with a RBBB configuration. The rhythm strip below illustrates a second hint: the premature P often is hidden in the T of the prior cycle.

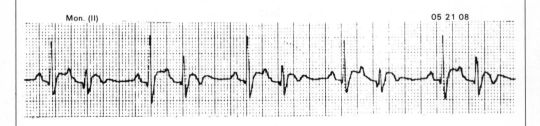

Thus, when a premature QRS is encountered, one must ask: "Is it preceded by a premature P?" And to find the premature P, one must inspect the prior T.

---

34. Study the strip in frame 26. Note the T prior to each premature QRS. These T waves are altered because they include

_____ .

a premature P.

35. There is one more feature of an APC. A premature stimulus from an atrial ectopic focus will discharge the sinus node along with the remainder of the atrial cells.

    The **rhythm of the sinus node usually is upset** by an APC.

36. An APC discharges the sinus node along with the remainder of the atrial tissue.

    Therefore, an APC

    _____ does not

    _____ does   *does*

    disturb the rhythm of the sinus node.

PAUSE FOLLOWING APC NOT COMPENSATORY

37. The pause following a premature beat is compensatory if it is long enough to compensate for the prematurity of the extrasystole. If there is a compensatory pause, the beat following the extrasystole occurs at the expected time. The meaning of a compensatory pause is this: If a compensatory pause is present, the premature beat did not interrupt the rhythmic discharge of the sinus node.

38. The pause following an APC usually is

    _____ compensatory.

    _____ less than compensatory.   *less than compensatory
                                                      (for the APC discharged*

    _____ more than compensatory.   *the sinus node).*

39.

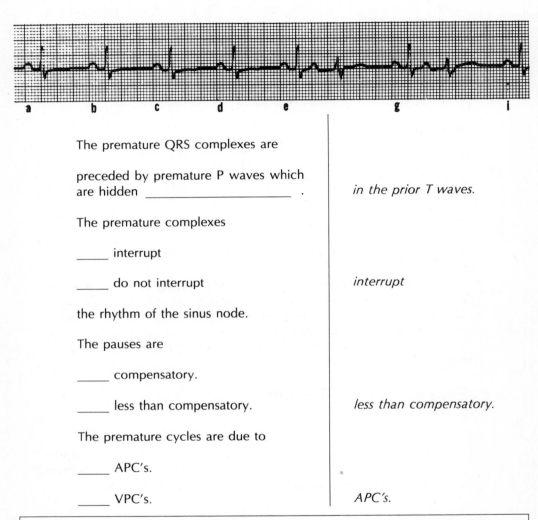

The premature QRS complexes are

preceded by premature P waves which
are hidden _____ .   *in the prior T waves.*

The premature complexes

_____ interrupt

_____ do not interrupt   *interrupt*

the rhythm of the sinus node.

The pauses are

_____ compensatory.

_____ less than compensatory.   *less than compensatory.*

The premature cycles are due to

_____ APC's.

_____ VPC's.   *APC's.*

40. An ectopic impulse arising in the atria generally discharges the sinus node.
Therefore, APC's usually are followed by a pause which is less than compensatory.

However, this is *not* an ironclad rule for distinguishing APC's from VPC's.

41. Five characteristics of an APC are:

1. _____

_____

_____

2. _____

_____

_____

3. _____

_____

_____

4. _____

_____

_____

5. _____

_____

_____

1. *P wave premature to the basic rhythm.*

2. *P wave configuration different* **(usually).** May be hidden in prior T.

3. *PR interval longer than, shorter than, or same as in the sinus cycles.*

4. *QRS usually has same configuration as other supraventricular cycles. However, aberrant ventricular conduction common, causing anomalous QRS, often of RBBB variety.*

5. *Ectopic impulse discharges sinus node prematurely, disturbing rhythm of the sinus node. Therefore, APC is followed by a pause which is not compensatory* **(usually).**

42. Proceed through a standard inquiry to determine if a premature QRS is of ventricular or supraventricular origin.

Feature of Premature QRS	Origin	
	Ventricular	*Supraventricular*
Narrow and the same as in the sinus cycles.	No	Yes
Anomalous (broader and ''different'').	Yes	No (unless aberrant ventricular conduction present)
Preceded by premature P.	No	Yes (but P may be hidden)
Interrupts the rhythm of the sinus node; subsequent pause is less than compensatory.	No (usually)	Yes (usually)
Subsequent pause is compensatory.	Yes (usually)	No (usually)

JUNCTIONAL PREMATURE COMPLEXES

43. Proceed now to the other focus of ectopic supraventricular rhythms, the A-V junction.

The junctional tissue may serve as a focus for escape rhythms, premature beats, or tachycardia.

44. Spread of a depolarization wave through the A-V junction produces only a small voltage; it does not produce a deflection on the ordinary ECG. If an impulse arises in the junction, we won't know about it until it breaks out into the atria (producing a P wave) or into the ventricles (producing a QRS complex).

Headward spread from junction toward atria is called **retrograde conduction.** Footward spread from junction toward ventricles is called **antegrade conduction.**

Whether P comes before QRS, after QRS or simultaneous with QRS depends on the relative speed of retrograde and antegrade conduction. Unless P is hidden in QRS, the PR or RP interval usually is short (0.10 sec. or less).

45. This junctional premature impulse found that antegrade conduction to the ventricles was rapid, retrograde conduction to the atria was slow. You will expect to find

_____ P prior to QRS.

_____ QRS prior to P.

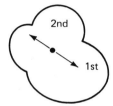

QRS prior to P.

LADDER DIAGRAM OF A JUNCTIONAL PREMATURE IMPULSE
WHICH TRAVELLED UPWARD AND DOWNWARD
SIMULTANEOUSLY BUT REACHED THE VENTRICLES FIRST.

46.

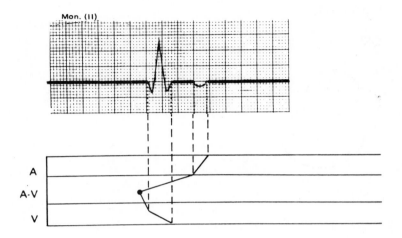

An impulse was initiated in the A-V junction. This spike is not demonstrable in the routine ECG. Antegrade conduction was rapid. It didn't take long to reach the ventricles and produce a QRS complex.

Retrograde conduction was slow. There was considerable delay before it reached the atrial muscle and produced a P wave. P was negative because the depolarization wave was spreading in a headward direction, away from the positive electrode.

---

47. From the A-V junctional apparatus the impulse may travel both directions. If it reaches the atria before the ventricles, the headward-spreading atrial depolarization will produce a negative P wave soon followed by QRS (**JPC with prior activation of the atria**).

If the depolarization wave reaches the ventricles prior to the atria, QRS occurs first, soon followed by an inverted P (**JPC with prior activation of the ventricles**).

If the depolarization wave reaches the atria and ventricles simultaneously, the inverted P is hidden in the larger QRS complex (**JPC with simultaneous depolarization of atria and ventricles**).

48.

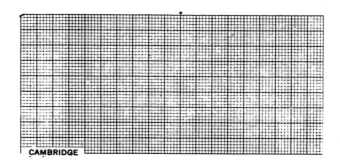

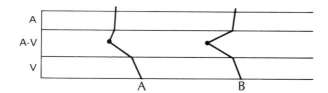

Review "Use of Ladder Diagram," page 84. Draw the ECG suggested by the ladder diagrams.

(A) represents a **junctional impulse with prior activation of the atria.**

(B) represents a **junctional impulse with simultaneous activation of ventricles and atria.**

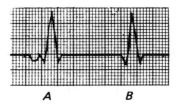

49.

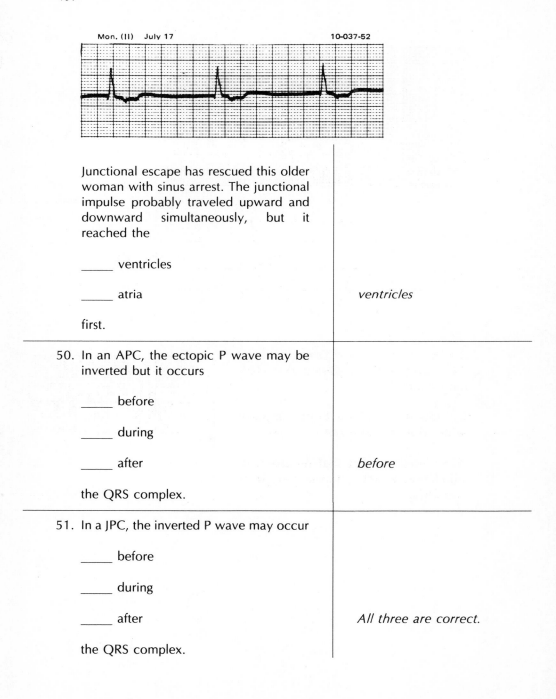

Mon. (II)   July 17   10-037-52

Junctional escape has rescued this older woman with sinus arrest. The junctional impulse probably traveled upward and downward simultaneously, but it reached the

_____ ventricles

_____ atria   *ventricles*

first.

50. In an APC, the ectopic P wave may be inverted but it occurs

_____ before

_____ during

_____ after   *before*

the QRS complex.

51. In a JPC, the inverted P wave may occur

_____ before

_____ during

_____ after   *All three are correct.*

the QRS complex.

52.

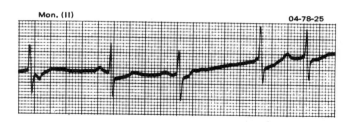

Mon. (II)   04-78-25

QRS configuration indicates that the first
complex is supraventricular. It is not an
APC, for the P occurs after QRS. This is
a JPC with prior activation of the

_____ atria.

_____ ventricles.   *ventricles.*

53. If a premature P is inverted and the PR interval is normal or short, distinguishing between an APC and a JPC usually is not possible in a single
monitoring lead.

54.

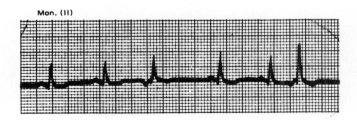

Mon. (II)

There are two inverted, premature P waves. Either might be junctional. However, they could be APC's.

Note the R-R intervals. Why is the second premature complex associated with aberrant ventricular conduction?

_____

_____

The second APC occurs so early, a portion of the His-Purkinje system is still refractory.

A RECAPITULATION

55. A junctional premature complex is characterized by:

1. Inverted P preceding, hidden in, or following QRS.

2. Short PR or RP interval.

3. QRS duration and configuration same as in the sinus cycles (unless aberrant ventricular conduction occurs).

56.

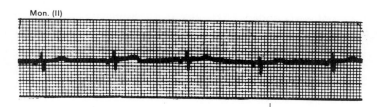

Mon. (II)

The A-V junction may replace the sinus node as a pacemaker. Junctional rhythm is illustrated in this tracing.

The P wave is _____.

inverted.

The PR interval is _____ sec.

0.08

57.

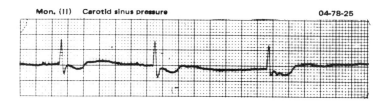

Mon. (II)   Carotid sinus pressure   04-78-25

Carotid sinus pressure slowed the sinus node so much that junctional escape occurred (QRS No. 3). In the escape cycle there was prior activation of the

_____ atria.

_____ ventricles.

ventricles.

SUMMARY—CHAPTER IX

1. If P waves are not well defined, often we cannot distinguish between atrial and junctional origin of an arrhythmia, and simply term it "supraventricular."

2. Narrow QRS complexes are of supraventricular origin.

3. Features of an APC:

    a. Premature P, usually of different configuration.
    b. PR short, normal or long. Sometimes the premature P is non-conducted (blocked).
    c. QRS narrow and the same as those of sinus origin (unless aberrant ventricular conduction is present).
    d. Premature P interrupts rhythm of the sinus node; pause usually less than compensatory.

4. Features of a JPC:

    a. Premature, inverted P occurs before, after or within the QRS.
    b. QRS narrow and the same (unless aberrant conduction present).
    c. Pause usually less than compensatory.

PROBLEMS — CHAPTER IX

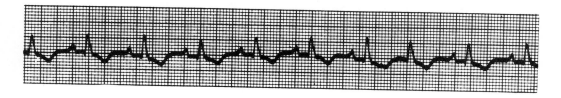

1. Summarize your description of the above strip. _____

_____

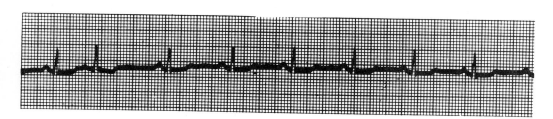

2. Summarize your description of the above strip. _____

_____

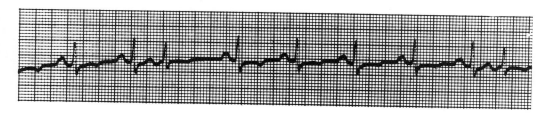

3. What is the premature cycle? _____

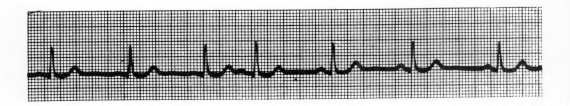

4. What is the premature cycle? _____

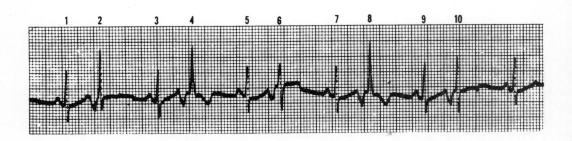

5. Describe this arrhythmia. _____

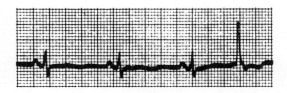

6. What is the premature cycle? _____

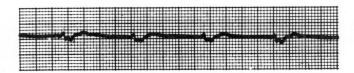

7. What is this arrhythmia? _____

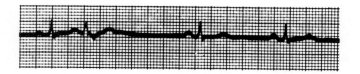

8. What is the premature beat? _____

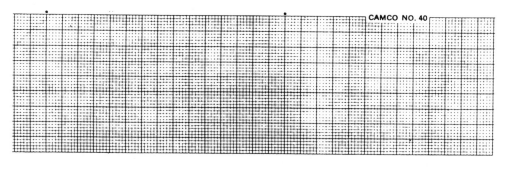

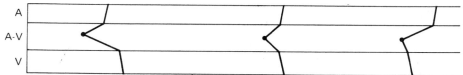

9. Sketch the P-QRS complexes for each of the junctional (A-V nodal) complexes diagrammed.

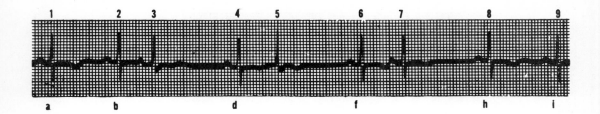

10. What sort of premature complexes are these? _____

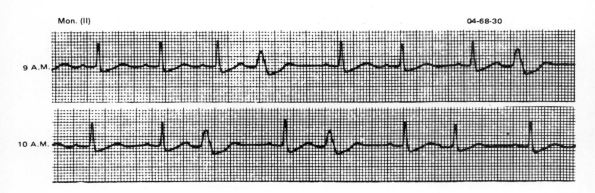

11. Routine lidocaine treatment for VPC's was not helpful in this patient with numerous premature complexes which were broad and "different." What are they? _____

chapter 10

atrial and junctional tachycardia (supraventricular tachycardia)

---

1.   CHARACTERISTICS OF ATRIAL TACHYCARDIA

1. Rate is 140–220/min. and remains constant hour after hour.

2. Rhythm is regular, often perfectly regular. However, when it occurs in brief paroxysms, atrial rhythm is likely to be irregular. Furthermore, block of some P waves may cause ventricular irregularity.

3. QRS duration 0.10 sec. or less unless AVC is present.

4. P wave configuration different from that present during sinus rhythm. (P usually hidden.)

Each of these characteristics has its exceptions and modifications.

---

2. The depolarization wave which starts in the atria is distributed to the ventricles by the rapidly conducting His-Purkinje system.

   If the ventricles are activated from above, the QRS duration will be

   _____ narrow

   _____ broad   *narrow*

   unless abnormal ventricular conduction is present (BBB or aberration).

3. QRS may be broad despite a supraventricular focus if there is bundle branch block or _____ .

   aberrant ventricular conduction.

4. In atrial tachycardia, the focus is different, outside the sinus node. The general direction of atrial activation is different.

   Thus, P wave configuration during atrial tachycardia differs from that during sinus rhythms.

5. In atrial tachycardia, four of the expected characteristics are

   1. _____

   2. _____

   3. _____

   4. _____

1. regular ventricular rhythm

2. ventricular rate 140–220/min.

3. narrow QRS

4. P waves different, or hidden

6.

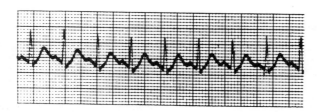

If the rate were much faster or the PR much longer, this P wave might be hard to see, for it would be hidden in ____

_____ .

the prior T wave.

7.

Mon. (II)

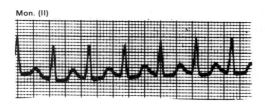

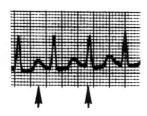

Make arrows to indicate where the P wave might be located.

P could be hidden in T or in QRS.

8. Often one is unable to determine that the T hides a P until after the paroxysm is terminated. Only now is T unadulterated with P.

9. Carotid sinus massage either terminates atrial tachycardia, or has no effect.

CAROTID SINUS MASSAGE

BEFORE 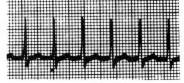 AFTER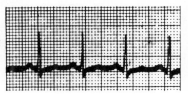

When sinus rhythm returns after carotid sinus massage, note the subtle change in T configuration. During tachycardia, P probably was hidden in T.

SUPRAVENTRICULAR TACHYCARDIA

10. More often than not, the P wave in atrial tachycardia is hidden and it might be safer to use the vague, noncommittal term, **supraventricular tachycardia.** This indicates we do not know whether the ectopic focus was atrial or junctional.

11.

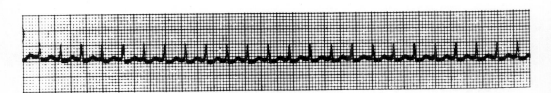

What label would you use for this tachy-cardia?

Supraventricular tachycardia, probably atrial.

12. Supraventricular tachycardia may produce a broad QRS due to **aberrant ventricular conduction.**

A RECAPITULATION FROM CHAPTER VIII

1. AVC most often is due to delay in the right bundle system.

2. When there is right bundle delay, the last areas to be depolarized are in the right ventricle.

3. The right ventricle is anterior.

4. The last forces of ventricular depolarization then point toward the front of the chest.

5. When the positive electrode is over the right ventricle (Lead V1 or MCL-1), the last part of QRS is positive when AVC is due to delay in the right bundle.

13.

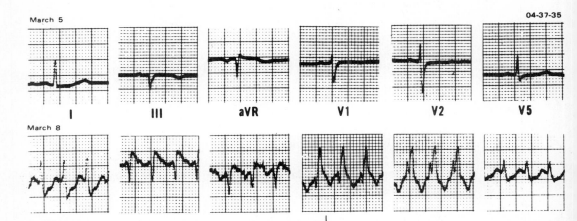

March 5

04-37-35

I   III   aVR   V1   V2   V5

March 8

When the rate became fast, this woman developed delay in activation of the right ventricle. Then there was a broad QRS with the last QRS forces pointing toward the V1 and V2 electrode positions. (Thus there is an RSR' in the right chest lead.)

This is a common finding with _____
_____ .

aberrant ventricular conduction.

14. Following are some characteristics of atrial tachycardia. Which characteristics always are present?

1. P wave abnormal.

2. Rate 140–220/min.

3. Rhythm perfectly regular.

4. Rate stays precisely the same, hour after hour.

5. QRS duration 0.10 sec. or less in the monitoring lead.

1. Not always. P often is hidden in prior T or QRS.
2. Not always.
3. No. Brief spells in particular often are a little irregular.
4. Not always.
5. No. Aberration is common, or patient may have preceding BBB.

ATRIAL TACHYCARDIA WITH BLOCK

15. When the rate is fast enough, the junctional tissue may not be able to recuperate fully between cycles; as a result A-V conduction may be prolonged or blocked.

    Block may produce an A-V ratio of 2:1, 3:1, 4:1, etc., or the A-V ratio may be variable.

16.

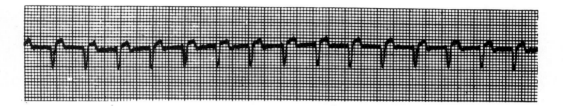

The atrial rate is _____ /min.	*146*
The ventricular rate is _____ /min.	*146*
The ratio of P waves to QRS complexes is _____.	*1:1*
The A-V ratio is _____.	*1:1*
This is atrial tachycardia with _____ A-V conduction.	*1:1*

17. **Physiologic block** at the A-V junction protects the ventricles from an excess rate of bombardment when the atrial rate is excessive.

18.

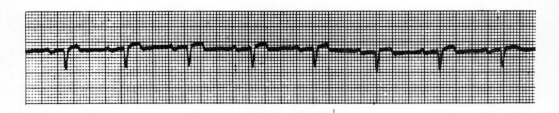

This is an example of atrial tachycardia in the same patient represented in frame 16.

The atrial rate is _____ /min.   *156*

The ventricular rate is _____ /min.   *78*

The ratio of P waves to QRS complexes
is _____.   *2:1*

The A-V ratio is _____.   *2:1*

This demonstrates _____ A-V con-   *2:1*
duction.

---

19. Atrial tachycardia with 2:1 block often is due to excessive digitalis effect.

20. Make ladder diagrams to illustrate events before and after 2:1 block developed in the patient shown above in frames 16 and 18.

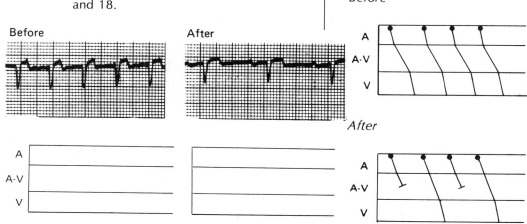

21. **Distinction between atrial and junctional tachycardia** is difficult because the crucial determinant, the P wave, often is hidden.

    In atrial tachycardia, P frequently is hidden in the prior T or QRS.

    In junctional tachycardia, P may be buried in QRS or truly absent due to failure of atrial activation (retrograde V-A block).

22. Use of the term **supraventricular tachycardia** indicates it is not possible to be more specific in identifying a tachycardia with normal QRS duration.

    Although sinus tachycardia, atrial flutter, and atrial fibrillation are of supraventricular origin, their specific diagnosis usually is possible.

    Thus, use of the **noncommittal term supraventricular tachycardia generally indicates inability to distinguish between ectopic atrial and A-V junctional origin.**

23. Abnormal P configuration and normal QRS duration would be expected

    _____ in both atrial and junctional tachycardia.

    _____ only with atrial tachycardia.

    _____ only with junctional tachycardia.

in both atrial and junctional tachycardia.

---

24. **Junctional tachycardia is similar to atrial tachycardia** in that:

    1. QRS duration is normal (unless aberrant ventricular conduction is present).

    2. Rhythm is quite regular, usually.

    3. Rate is constant over a period of time, usually.

    However, **junctional tachycardia differs from atrial tachycardia** in that:

    1. P waves are inverted (when the lead axis is similar to leads II, III or aVF), indicating retrograde activation of the atria.

    2. P waves come shortly before or after QRS, or are buried within the QRS complexes.

    3. Rate usually is below 150 per minute.

25.

Lead II

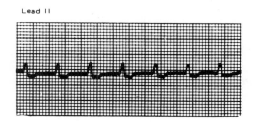

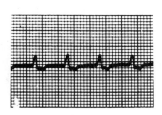

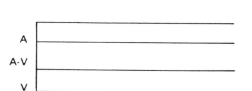

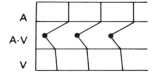

Sketch the mechanism on the ladder diagram.

In this junctional tachycardia,

the P wave direction is _____.   *inverted.*

The R-P interval is _____ sec.   *0.06*

---

26. Since the normal rate of a junctional pacemaker is 40–60/min., sometimes
a junctional rhythm at a rate of 80 is called junctional **"tachycardia."** We
prefer to reserve use of the word tachycardia for rates in excess of 100/min.
Perhaps a junctional rhythm at a rate of 80 could be called **"accelerated
junctional rhythm."**

CLINICAL SIGNIFICANCE OF ACCELERATED JUNCTIONAL RHYTHMS

27. Digitalis toxicity can accelerate a junctional focus.

Excess digitalis effect is suspect whenever a junctional focus shows abnormal automaticity, resulting in a junctional rate above 60/min.

SUMMARY—CHAPTER X

1. Atrial tachycardia usually is regular at a rate of 140–220/min.

2. P waves are of different configuration, but usually are hidden.

3. QRS is narrow unless aberrant conduction occurs.

4. Because junctional tachycardia usually cannot be distinguished from atrial tachycardia, the term supraventricular tachycardia is useful.

PROBLEMS—CHAPTER X

Most cases of atrial tachycardia have a rate above 180. However, there is a grey zone between 140 and 180/min. where the differentiation between sinus tachycardia and atrial tachycardia may be aided by the following comparison:

Sinus Tachycardia	Atrial Tachycardia
1. P configuration same as during normal sinus rhythm.	P configuration _____.
2. Gradual acceleration to the rapid rate.	Rapid rate usually starts _____.
3. Gradual deceleration.	Deceleration usually is _____.
4. Sitting, rolling, coughing, straining usually produce some variation in R-R interval.	The rate (R-R interval) is usually _____ over a period of hours, despite maneuvers which modify vagal tone.
5. Carotid sinus massage may cause temporary slowing.	Carotid massage produces _____.

A	
A-V	
V	

2. A 48-year-old man developed congestive failure three days after myocardial infarction. Thorough digitalization helped somewhat, but major improvement did not occur until I.V. diuretics were used. On the sixth day, tachycardia, hypotension, and cold extremities suddenly developed.

Use the ladder diagram to indicate the mechanism of this tachycardia.

chapter 11

atrial flutter

1.   CHARACTERISTICS OF ATRIAL FLUTTER

Atrial rhythm regular.

Atrial rate 250–375, and most often about 300/min.

Sawtooth appearance of flutter waves. In some leads, the baseline constantly is in motion.

Ventricular rate and rhythm variable, determined by degree of A-V block.

Conduction of every 2nd or 4th flutter wave produces regular rhythm at rate of 150 or 75/min.

Variable conduction may produce irregular ventricular rhythm.

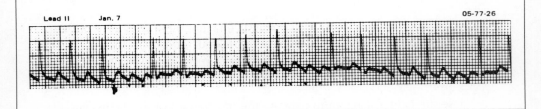

Lead II   Jan. 7   05-77-26

2. In atrial flutter, the atrial rate is about
_____ /min.

	300

3.

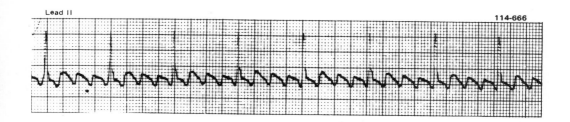

Lead II   114-666

The interval between the flutter waves is
_____ small squares.

five

The atrial rate is _____ /min.

$$300 \quad 5\overline{)1500}^{\,300}$$

The ventricular rate is _____ /min.

75

---

4. Atrial flutter waves often appear sawtoothed, due to continuous motion of the baseline. Whether or not this appearance is noted depends on:

   1. Lead axis. (It is seen best when the axis is similar to leads II, III, and aVF.)

   2. Ventricular rate. (Closely spaced QRS complexes will obscure the smaller flutter waves.)

---

5. Thus, to find flutter waves:

   1. Obtain different leads (II, II, aVF, esophageal, or right atrial).

   2. Slow the ventricular rate by vagal stimulation. (A cough, the Valsalva maneuver, carotid massage, or a change of position may be useful.)

6.

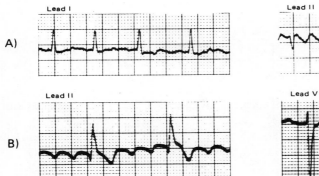

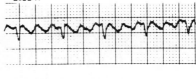

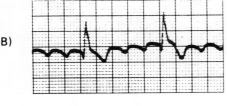

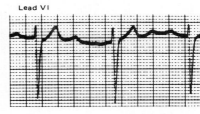

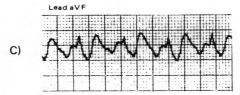

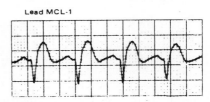

Multiple leads are necessary in a search for flutter waves. In the three cases above, flutter waves are

	present in lead	absent in lead	*present*	*absent*
Case A	____	____	*II*	*I*
Case B	____	____	*II*	*V1*
Case C	____	____	obscure in both leads, but suspected in aVF	

A GOOD RULE TO REMEMBER

7. When troubled or puzzled, divide the suspected P-P interval in half.

   Then ask, "Could another P be hidden halfway between the obvious P waves?"

8.

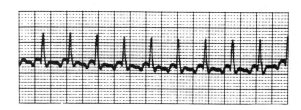

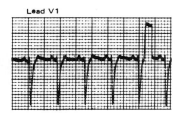

Lead V1

Label the suspected P waves.

The P-P interval appears to be _____ sec.

0.36 sec.

Half the obvious P-P interval is _____.

0.18 sec.

Is there a hidden atrial wave half way between the obvious waves? _____

Yes

The true atrial rate is _____ /min. and this is consistent with _____ .

350/min.
atrial flutter.

---

9. Flutter must be suspected when uniform undulations occur with an interval of 4 or 5 or 6 small squares. The atrial rate generally is 375 to 250/min.

---

10. Vagal stimulation may slow the ventricular rate and uncover flutter waves.

11.

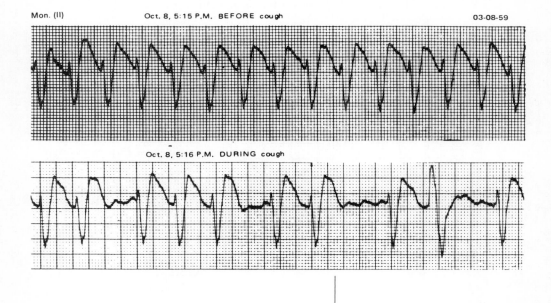

Mon. (II)　　　　Oct. 8, 5:15 P.M. BEFORE cough　　　　03-08-59

Oct. 8, 5:16 P.M. DURING cough

Cough slowed the ventricular rate momentarily, revealing regular undulations at a rate of about _____ .

300/min.

This suggests the diagnosis of _____ .

atrial flutter.

QRS is broad due to bundle branch block or _____

_____

aberrant ventricular conduction.

FEATURES OF THE ATRIAL WAVES IN ATRIAL FLUTTER

12. Thus far we have discussed features of the atrial mechanism with atrial flutter.

1. Atrial rhythm regular.

2. Atrial rate about 300.

3. Flutter waves often hidden by QRS complexes, or seen only in certain leads.

QRS FEATURES IN ATRIAL FLUTTER

13. 1. As in all supraventricular rhythms, QRS is narrow unless bundle branch block or aberrant ventricular conduction is present.

    2. The A-V junctional apparatus seldom can conduct more than 250 impulses a minute; therefore some degree of A-V block usually is present.

    3. The ratio of atrial to ventricular complexes (A-V ratio) commonly is 2:1 or 4:1. If atrial rate is 300, a regular 2:1 A-V ratio will produce a regular ventricular rhythm at a rate of 150. A regular 4:1 A-V ratio will produce a regular ventricular rhythm at a rate of 75. However, A-V conduction may vary from moment to moment, resulting in an irregular ventricular rhythm.

14. Most often, alternate flutter waves are conducted, the A-V ratio is 2:1 and the ventricular rhythm is regular at a rate of about 150/minute.

15.

Mon. (II)

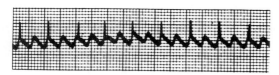

The atrial rate is _____ /min.   *336*

The ventricular rate is _____ /min.   *168*

The ratio, atrial rate: ventricular rate, equals _____.

2:1 (Often this is called 2:1 A-V conduction.)

16. When the ventricular rhythm is regular at a rate of about 150/min., always think of atrial flutter with 2:1 conduction.

17.

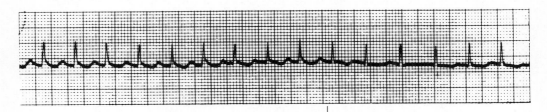

The ventricular rate is _____ per minute.

146

Ventricular rhythm is _____ regular _____ irregular

regular

When the ventricular rhythm is regular at a rate of about 150/min., always think of _____ .

atrial flutter with 2:1 conduction

Two things which might help to demonstrate the underlying atrial mechanism would be (see frame 6):

1. get different leads

1. _____

2. make a record during cough, straining, turning or carotid massage.

2. _____

---

18. Atrial flutter waves occur so rapidly that the junctional apparatus can conduct only a portion of them to the ventricles. Some flutter waves, victims of **concealed partial A-V penetration,** get jammed in the gateway and do not reach the ventricles.

Flutter waves which do not reach the ventricles are **blocked.**

19.

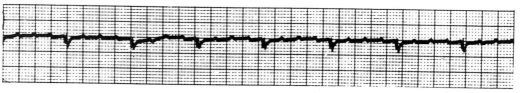

The atrial rate is _____ /min.	*290*
The ventricular rate is _____ /min.	*73*
The ratio of atrial to ventricular complexes is _____.	*4:1*
This is an example of _____ A-V block.	*4:1 (Often this is called 4:1 A-V conduction.)*

20. When the ventricular rhythm is regular at a rate of about 75, think of atrial flutter with 4:1 block.

When the ventricular rhythm is regular at a rate of about 150, think of atrial flutter with 2:1 block.

When the ventricular rhythm is irregular at a rate of 60–160, think of atrial flutter with variable block.

For that matter, always think of atrial flutter.

21.

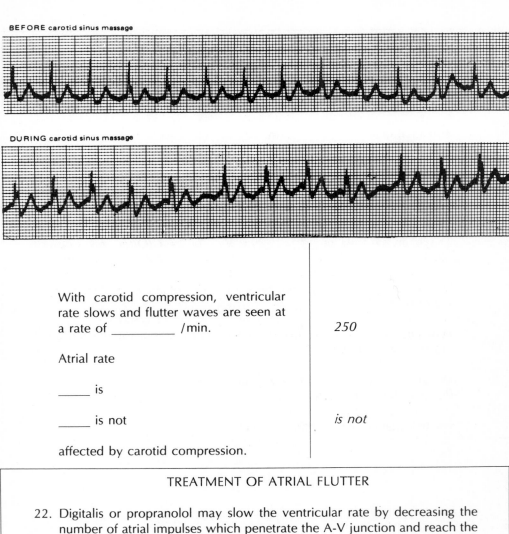

BEFORE carotid sinus massage

DURING carotid sinus massage

With carotid compression, ventricular rate slows and flutter waves are seen at a rate of _____ /min.

250

Atrial rate

_____ is

_____ is not

is not

affected by carotid compression.

TREATMENT OF ATRIAL FLUTTER

22. Digitalis or propranolol may slow the ventricular rate by decreasing the number of atrial impulses which penetrate the A-V junction and reach the ventricles.

Cardioversion often is used to terminate atrial flutter.

---

23. If digitalization suddenly changes the rate of a regular tachycardia from 150 to 75/min., the underlying mechanism may be _____.

atrial flutter.

24.

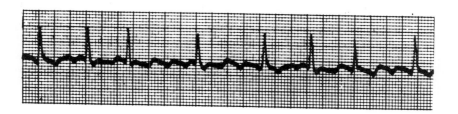

This is an example of atrial flutter with variable A-V block (often called variable A-V conduction) following digitalization. Note that there are two or three or four flutter waves for each QRS complex.

25. In frame 24, the atrial rate is _____ /min.	*260*
The ventricular rate is _____ /min.	*88*
The A-V ratio is _____ constant.	
_____ variable.	*variable.*
26. If the atrial rate is 300 per minute, what is the ventricular rate when there is	
2:1 block? ____ /min.	*150*
3:1 block? ____ /min.	*100*
4:1 block? ____ /min.	*75*

QUINIDINE EFFECT

27. Quinidine enhances A-V conduction and slows the atrial flutter rate. As successive doses of quinidine are given, the atrial rate may fall to a level which permits 1:1 conduction.

28. Complete the chart to indicate what might happen to the ventricular rate as successive doses of quinidine are given to a patient with atrial flutter.

Quinidine Effect	Atrial Rate	A-V Ratio	Ventricular Rate	Ventricular Rate
None	300	2:1	____/min.	*150*
Slight	280	2:1	____/min.	*140*
Moderate	220	2:1	____/min.	*110*
Substantial	190	1:1	____/min.	*190*

29.

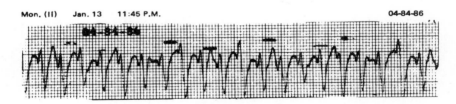

Mon. (II)   Jan. 13   11:45 P.M.   04-84-86

A middle-aged man with atrial flutter suddenly collapsed after his eighth dose of quinidine. What is the ventricular rate? _____ /min.

244/min.

We can't make a definite diagnosis from the rhythm strip, but what mechanism should be considered? _____

Quinidine may have slowed the flutter rate until 1:1 conduction was possible.

ALWAYS SUSPECT ATRIAL FLUTTER

30. **Failure to recognize atrial flutter** is a common, serious error in ECG arrhythmia diagnosis.

A **diagnosis** must be *thought of* before it can be *made*.

Treatment of a catastrophically rapid ventricular rate due to flutter can be simple and life-saving.

A **supraventricular tachycardia with** *regular* **ventricular rhythm** always raises the question of atrial flutter with 2:1 A-V conduction.

A **supraventricular tachycardia with** *irregular* **ventricular rhythm** always raises the question of atrial flutter with variable A-V conduction.

A **broad QRS tachycardia** with *regular* **ventricular rhythm** always raises the question of atrial flutter with aberration and 2:1 A-V conduction.

A **broad QRS tachycardia** with *irregular* **ventricular rhythm** always raises the question of atrial flutter with aberration and variable A-V conduction.

SUMMARY—CHAPTER XI

1. During atrial flutter atrial rhythm is regular at a rate of about 300/min.

2. Usually, the baseline constantly is in motion in some lead, producing a sawtooth appearance.

3. Ventricular rhythm often is regular at a rate one-half the atrial rate, namely, about 150/min.

4. Hidden flutter waves may be uncovered by slowing the ventricular rate (carotid compression or other vagal maneuver).

5. Digitalis and propranolol may slow the ventricular rate by impairing A-V conduction.

6. Quinidine may enhance A-V conduction. Also, it may reduce the flutter rate to a level which permits 1:1 conduction.

PROBLEMS—CHAPTER XI

1.

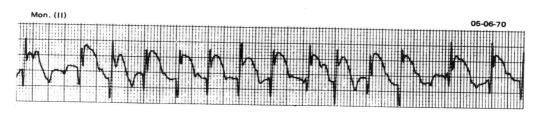

Mon. (II)   05-06-70

Atrial waves are obscured by the closely spaced, larger QRST deflections.
Therefore look closely where the R-R interval is longer.

The atrial rate is _____ /min. and the diagnosis is _____ .

2.

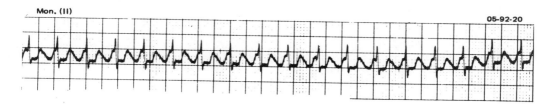

Mon. (II)   05-92-20

1. What is the atrial rate? _____
2. What is the ventricular rate? _____
3. What is the atrio-ventricular ratio? _____

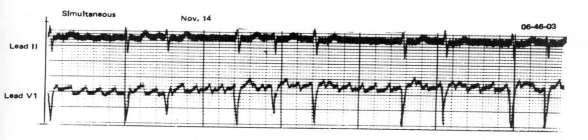

Simultaneous   Nov. 14   06-46-03

Lead II

Lead V1

3. Indicate the following:

1. Ventricular rate   _____ /min.
2. Atrial rate   _____ /min.
3. Do you see flutter waves in lead II?   _____
4. Do you see flutter waves in lead V1?   _____
5. Rhythm diagnosis   _____

4.

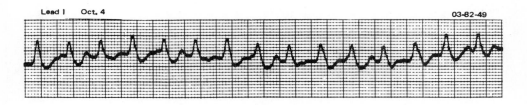

1. A regular rhythm with a rate of about 150/min. always requires consideration of _____ with 2:1 block.
2. The broad QRS could be related to the fast rate. If so, it might represent _____ conduction.

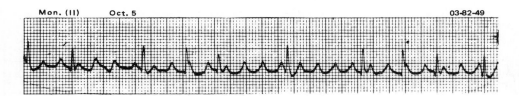

3. Digitalis has been given. This drug *(speeds) (impairs)* conduction through the A-V node.
4. Now the ventricular rate has slowed to _____ /min.

   The atrial rate is _____ /min.

5.

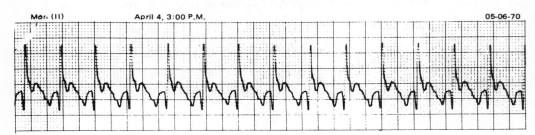

Hypotension, continuing pain, sweating, and pronounced apprehension were the chief problems of this 60-year-old man admitted two hours after the onset of crushing retrosternal discomfort radiating to the throat.

Examination: No cyanosis. Skin pale, damp and cool. Blood pressure 90/70. No murmur or rub. Bilateral basal rales.

1. Indicate the following:

   Ventricular rate   _____ /min.

   Ventricular rhythm   _____

2. Complete the following rule: "When the ventricular rhythm is regular at a rate of about 150, always think of . . ."

   _____

3. Complete the following rule: "When troubled or puzzled, divide the obvious P-P interval in half and ask . . ."

   _____

   _____

4. Complete the following:

   What is the P-P interval?   _____ sec.

   What is half the P-P interval?   _____ sec.

   Could another P wave be hidden halfway between the obvious P waves?

   _____

5. Demonstration of P waves often is crucial for rhythm diagnosis. List several procedures which might be done to help visualize P waves:

   _____

   _____

   _____

During Carotid Compression

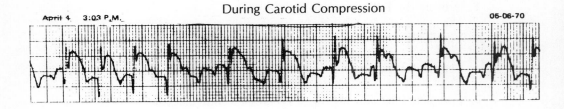

April 4   3:03 P.M.   05-06-70

6. Carotid compression is a form of vagal stimulation.

   (true) (false)   _____

7. Indicate the following:

   Atrial rate   _____ /min.

   Atrial rhythm   _____

   Rhythm diagnosis   _____

8. He deteriorated steadily. What treatments might be appropriate?

   _____

Following Cardioversion

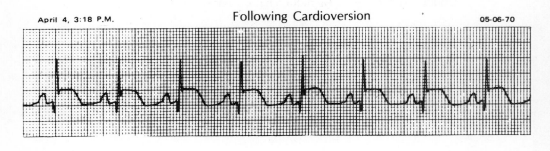

April 4, 3:18 P.M.   05-06-70

9. Rhythm diagnosis _____

chapter 12

atrial fibrillation

CHARACTERISTICS OF ATRIAL FIBRILLATION

1. During sinus rhythm a depolarization wave spreads smoothly through the atria, producing the P wave, then a coordinated contraction. In atrial fibrillation, uncoordinated, chaotic depolarization wavelets traverse a variable course from moment to moment. These wavelets traverse whatever fibers have recovered sufficiently to conduct, producing variable fibrillation waves on the ECG and a quivering atrial muscle.

   A. **Fibrillation waves** (sometimes called "f" waves) characteristically have the following features:

      1. Rate above 350/minute, and usually a good deal faster.

      2. Configuration varies from moment to moment.

      3. Rhythm irregular.

      4. Often inapparent or obscured by larger QRST waves.

   B. **Ventricular rhythm** is totally irregular (unless high degree A-V block is present).

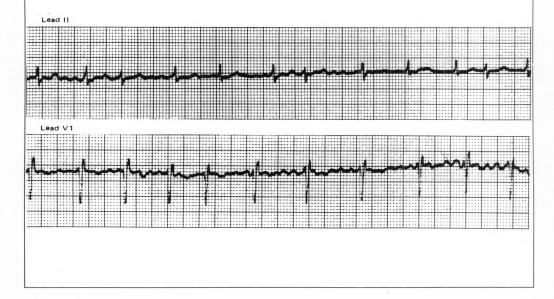

Lead II

Lead V1

2. Atrial *flutter* waves are uniform in configuration, regular in rhythm and occur at a rate of about _____ /min.

300

In atrial flutter, the ventricular rhythm may be irregular due to variable block, but more commonly there is a 2:1 A-V ratio with regular ventricular rhythm at a rate of about _____ , or a 4:1 ratio with a ventricular rate of about _____ .

150/min.

75/min.

3.

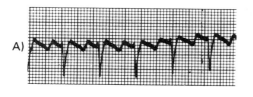

Tracing A shows atrial _____ .

flutter.

Tracing B shows atrial _____ .

fibrillation.

4. Atrial fibrillation waves vary in appearance from one moment to the next. (See frame 1, frame 3B and frame 6A.)

In the tracing below, note the baseline just before and just after the first QRS complex.

MCL-1

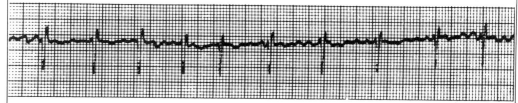

5.

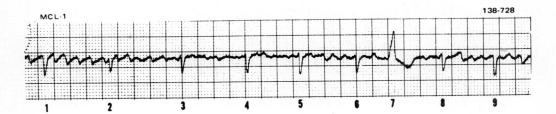

MCL-1   138-728

1   2   3   4   5   6   7   8   9

In this record there is marked variation in appearance of the fibrillation waves from moment to moment. The contour is typical of atrial fibrillation during R-R intervals 3-4 and 4-5. Intervals 1-2 and 8-9 have a sawtooth baseline suggesting _____.

atrial flutter.

6.

Lead VI

A)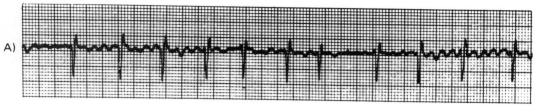

Lead VI

B)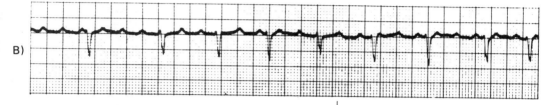

Tracing A shows atrial waves of variable contour at a rate of about 450/min. This is _____.

atrial fibrillation.

Tracing B shows atrial waves of uniform contour at a rate of about 242/min. This is _____.

atrial flutter.

7.

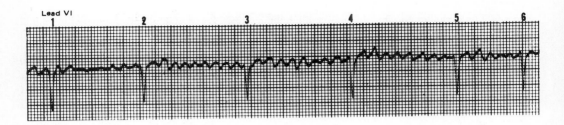

Lead VI

Atrial waves in this strip have the following characteristics of atrial fibrillation:

1. Rate is above 350/min.

2. Atrial rhythm is irregular.

3. Configuration varies from one "f" wave to the next.

4. _____

_____

Configuration changes from moment to moment. Compare the undulations between cycles 1 and 2, 3 and 4, 5 and 6.

FIBRILLATION TERMINOLOGY

8. Fibrillation waves may be **fine** (between cycles 1 and 2 of frame 7) or **coarse** (after cycle 2). But the important feature to remember is that configuration often varies from moment to moment. A poor term is **flutter-fibrillation,** sometimes used when a sawtooth pattern comes and goes. (See frames 5 and 7.)

9. Lead V1 or the monitoring lead MCL-1 may show fibrillation waves better than lead II or Mon. (II).

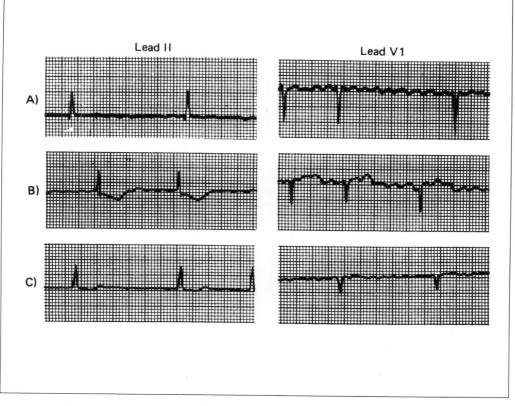

10. This patient has no apparent atrial activity.

What can you suggest? _____   *Try MCL-1.*

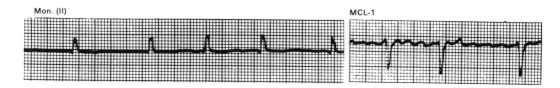

11. Invisibility of fibrillation waves is only a minor technical problem if it can be remedied by obtaining a different point of view—a different lead axis.

However, a more difficult impediment to visualizing "f" waves is a rapid ventricular rate. Closely spaced QRST complexes overshadow the smaller fibrillation waves.

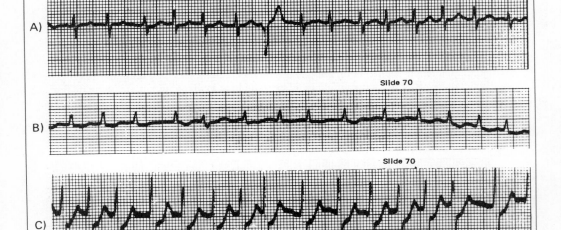

A)

Slide 70

B)

Slide 70

C)

12. Review illustrations in frames 10 and 11.

List two reasons why visualization of "f" waves cannot be relied upon to make the diagnosis of atrial fibrillation.

_____ See frame 10 lead Mon. (II)

_____ See frame 11.

Too small to see.

Rate so fast that "f" waves are hidden by larger QRST deflections.

13. Lacking clear "f" waves, a subtle clue to their presence may be otherwise unexplained **T wave variation.**

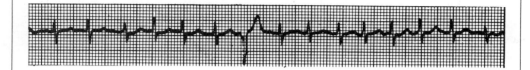

14. A second minor clue is slight **variation in QRS amplitude and configuration** from cycle to cycle.

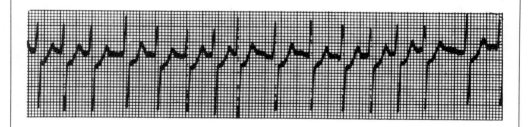

TOTALLY IRREGULAR VENTRICULAR RHYTHM

15. We have discussed the atrial pattern in atrial fibrillation. However, when "f" waves are hard to see, the major diagnostic clue is **total irregularity of ventricular rhythm.**

16.

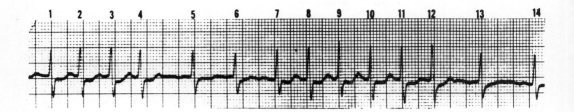

Tiny fibrillation waves may be present (See R-R intervals 6–7 and 12–13). However, the main clue regarding presence of atrial fibrillation is _____.

the absolutely irregular ventricular rhythm.

List additional clues which are consistent with the diagnosis of atrial fibrillation in this record:

T wave varies (compare nos. 12 and 13).

_____

QRS varies (compare nos. 6 and 9).

_____

---

17. In atrial fibrillation, the ventricular rhythm is totally irregular.

The rare exception is **atrial fibrillation with high degree A-V block.** If atrial impulses are blocked in the A-V junctional apparatus, a junctional or ventricular escape focus may have a chance to become manifest. An escape focus generally has a regular rhythm.

In atrial fibrillation with high degree A-V block, the ventricular rate ordinarily is slow (below 60 or 70/minute) and some of the R-R intervals are the same.

18.

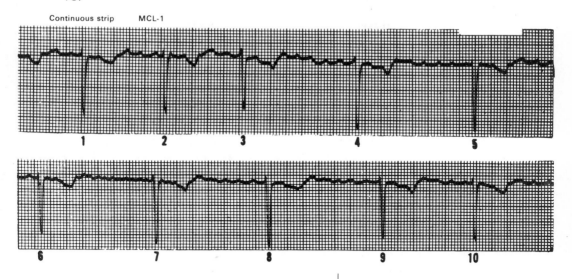

Continuous strip   MCL-1

Baseline undulations establish the diagnosis of atrial fibrillation. Measure the R-R intervals.

1–2 _____ sec.	6–7 _____ sec.	*1–2 1.04 sec.*	*6–7 1.44 sec.*
2–3 _____ sec.	7–8 _____ sec.	*2–3 1.00 sec.*	*7–8 1.44 sec.*
3–4 _____ sec.	8–9 _____ sec.	*3–4 1.44 sec.*	*8–9 1.44 sec.*
4–5 _____ sec.	9–10 _____ sec.	*4–5 1.46 sec.*	*9–10 1.20 sec.*
5–6 _____ sec.		*5–6 1.30 sec.*	

The diagnosis is atrial fibrillation with

_____

high degree A-V block.

The junctional escape focus has a discharge rate equivalent to an R-R interval of about _____ sec.

1.44

19.

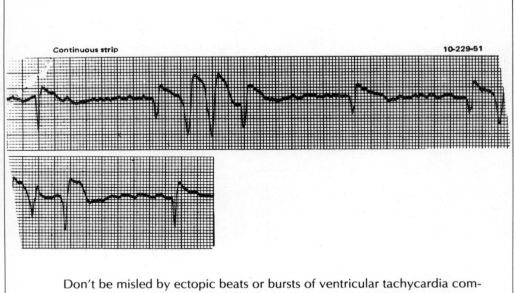

Continuous strip   10-229-51

Don't be misled by ectopic beats or bursts of ventricular tachycardia complicating atrial fibrillation with high degree A-V block. If the basic rate is slow and if many R-R intervals are nearly the same, suspect high degree A-V block.

20. As with all supraventricular arrhythmias, QRS duration is normal unless bundle branch block or aberration is present.

21.

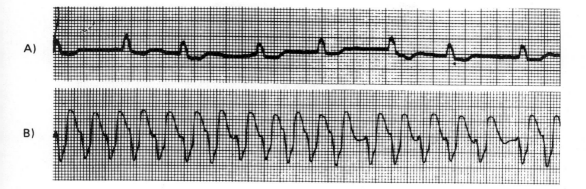

A)

B)

These records from different patients illustrate the same problem: broad QRS and irregular rhythm.

P waves are

_____ present.

_____ absent.   *absent.*

Fibrillation waves are

_____ seen.

_____ not seen.   *not seen.*

The rhythm of the atria may be _____ .   *atrial fibrillation.*

QRS is broad because of _____ .   *bundle branch block.*

Rhythm diagnosis is _____ .   *atrial fibrillation with bundle branch block.*

22.

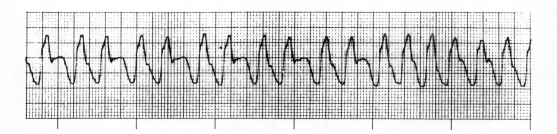

If atrial fibrillation causes a rapid ventricular rate, total irregularity may be overlooked. If QRS is broad, the resultant broad QRS tachycardia might be mistaken for _____ .

ventricular tachycardia.

23.

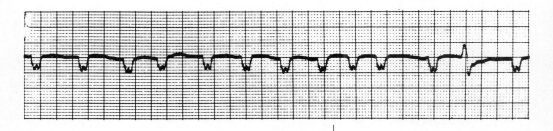

Atrial fibrillation waves are not apparent but we suspect this diagnosis because ventricular rhythm is _____ .

totally irregular.

24. Appearance of wide and decidedly **anomalous QRS complexes present the real diagnostic problem in atrial fibrillation.** Do these represent aberration or ventricular ectopic activity?

Lead II

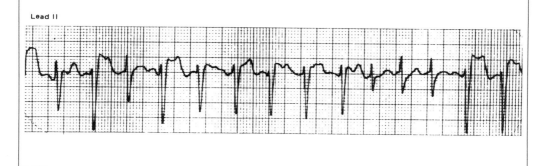

25. Fixed coupling and a pause following the anomalous beat favor ventricular ectopy.

Lead I   31079

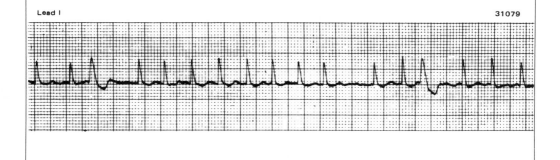

26.

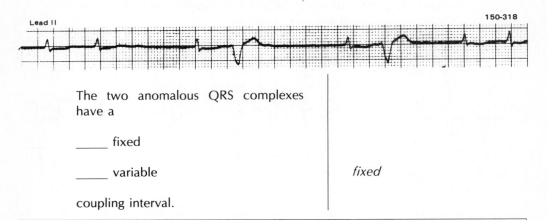

The two anomalous QRS complexes have a

_____ fixed

_____ variable   *fixed*

coupling interval.

---

27. Lead MCL-1 helps to distinguish ectopic from aberrant complexes.

RSR' IN MCL-1 FAVORS AVC

28. In lead V1 or MCL-1, aberration is favored if the anomalous complex shows features of RBBB. (Review Chapter VIII.) **Especially suggestive of aberration is an RSR' complex in V1 or MCL-1.**

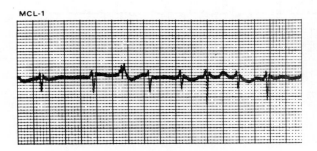

An RSR' configuration in MCL-1 is suggestive of aberration, not an inviolate rule.

29.

Mon. (II)

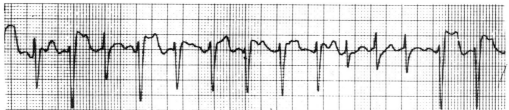

When a patient with atrial fibrillation has some anomalous QRS complexes, two possibilities must be considered:

1. _____

2. _____

ventricular ectopic complexes

aberrant conduction of supraventricular impulses

30. Experts may disagree on the cause of an anomalous QRS. The essential fact to remember is that there are two possibilities: ectopic origin and aberration.

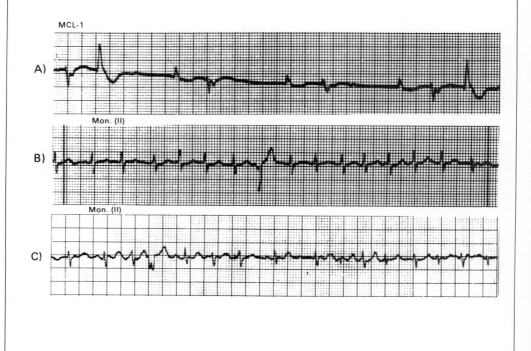

SUMMARY—CHAPTER XII

1. During atrial fibrillation atrial waves are irregular in contour and rhythm, at a rate above 350/min.

2. Fibrillation waves may be invisible in some leads, and may be obscured if ventricular rate is fast.

3. Ventricular rhythm is totally irregular.

4. Anomalous (broad and "different") QRS configuration may be due to aberrant conduction. The latter is favored by an RSR' pattern in MCL-1.

Rhythm strips for problem 1, page 179.

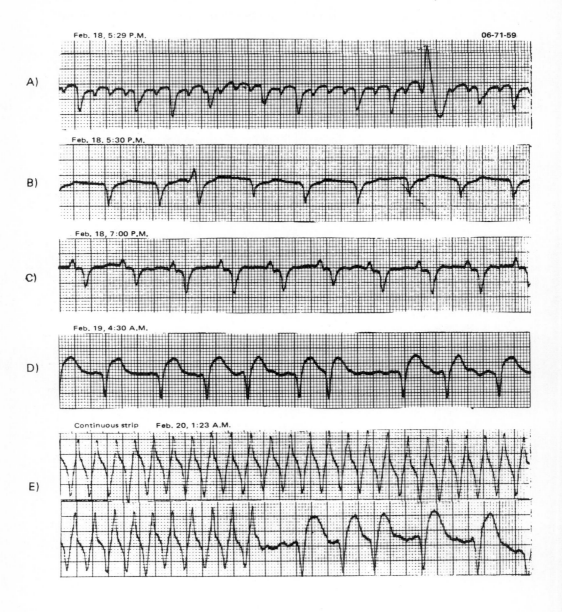

PROBLEMS—CHAPTER XII

1. This 71-year-old man had considerable congestive failure on February 18, his fifth day following a large infarction. Rhythm strips are shown on the facing page.

    A. Ventricular rhythm is *(regular) (irregular)*. Atrial mechanism is *(flutter) (fibrillation)*.
    B. Ventricular rhythm fundamentally is regular. QRS duration is *(normal) (prolonged)*. This rhythm is of *(supraventricular) (ventricular)* origin. The rhythm diagnosis is _____.
    C. Now the diagnosis is _____.
    D. Ventricular rhythm is irregular. Atrial mechanism is *(standstill) (flutter) (fibrillation)*.
    E. The two strips are continuous. Ventricular rate during the tachycardia is _____ /min. Immediately after the paroxysm are two or three atrial waves which look very much like _____.

    Perhaps the paroxysm was due to *(atrial flutter) (atrial fibrillation)* with 1:1 conduction.

2.

Lead III   73497

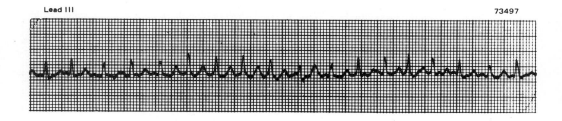

    1. The narrow QRS indicates that this arrhythmia is of *(supraventricular) (ventricular)* origin.
    2. The ventricular rhythm is *(regular) (irregular)*.
    3. The QRS complexes show *(slight) (no)* variation in contour and amplitude.
    4. Flutter waves are *(present) (absent)*.
    5. P waves are *(present) (absent)*.
    6. This completely irregular supraventricular tachycardia, without P waves or flutter waves, showing slight variation in QRS configuration, is an example of _____.

> ### REMEMBER
>
> If ventricular rate is rapid, don't expect to be able to see tiny fibrillation waves between the large QRS complexes.

3.

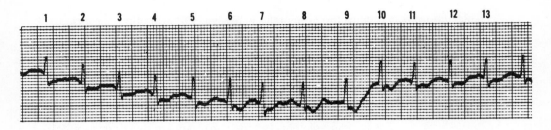

1. The ventricular rhythm is *(totally irregular)* *(basically regular)*.
2. Atrial fibrillation is *(a likely diagnosis)* *(unlikely)*.

4.

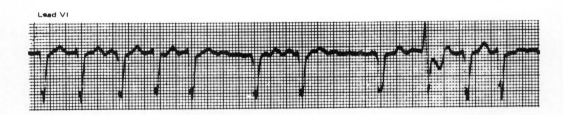

The rhythm diagnosis is _____

_____ .

5. A stuporous little old lady arrives shortly after her second fainting spell in recent weeks. Because of known angina and prior congestive failure, she is admitted to the Intensive Coronary Care Facility. In the depths of her purse is an enameled box with a good supply of six different sorts of pills.

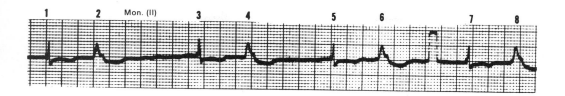

Describe her rhythm strip. _____

_____

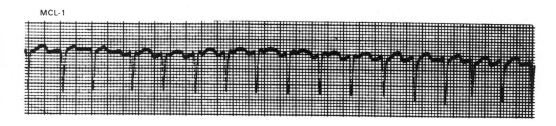

6. The rhythm diagnosis is:

_____

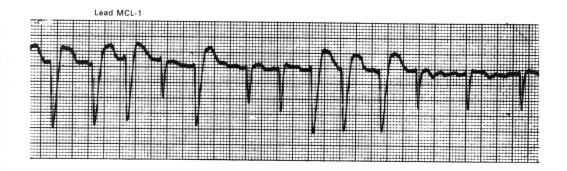

7. Do these clusters of broad QRS complexes demand urgent use of intravenous lidocaine?

_____ .

chapter 13

ventricular premature complexes

1. The same pathway of ventricular depolarization is used for all supraventricular impulses, whether of sinus, atrial or junctional origin.

2. If the pathway of ventricular depolarization is unchanged, QRS configuration will be

_____ the same.

_____ different.   *the same.*

3. QRS configuration is

_____ the same

_____ different   *the same*

for beats of sinus, atrial or A-V junctional origin.

4. A "different" configuration of QRS indicates a different depolarization pathway. A different pathway occurs if: The impulse has had ectopic origin within the ventricles; or there is aberrant conduction of a supraventricular impulse.

5. The depolarization wave which results in the QRS complex normally starts in the _____.

sinus node.

6. Where does the impulse arise in a VPC?

In the ventricle.

7. Full use of the His-Purkinje rapid transit system is reserved for depolarization waves commencing in the supraventricular tissue.

8. A depolarization wave of supraventricular origin gets aboard the His-Purkinje system and is distributed rapidly throughout the ventricles.

A depolarization wave of ventricular origin does not fully utilize the His-Purkinje system. It is distributed via the slowly conducting, ordinary muscle fibers.

9. The depolarization wave causing a VPC arises in the ventricles. It cannot utilize the His-Purkinje system. It is distributed slowly, via ordinary muscle fibers. The resultant QRS is

_____ broader

_____ narrower

broader

than a depolarization wave of supraventricular origin.

10. When the QRS complex is of supraventricular origin, QRS duration usually is 0.10 sec. or less in the monitoring lead. However, supraventricular origin may be associated with a broad QRS if BBB or aberrant ventricular conduction is present. (See Chapter VIII.)

11. Duration of a QRS complex of supraventricular origin usually is _____ sec. or less in a monitoring lead.

0.10

12. Duration of the QRS complex due to a VPC usually is _____ sec. or more in a monitoring lead.

0.11

13. Each lead provides a different vantage point from which to view the depolarization wave. Thus, with VPC's or with sinus beats, QRS duration may be different in different leads.

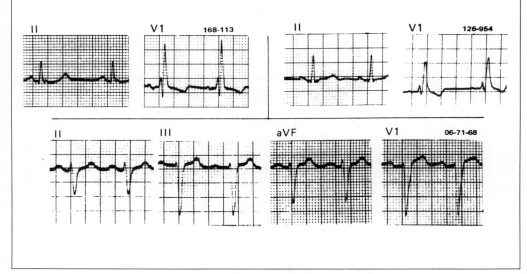

14. Frame 12 indicates that a VPC has a duration of 0.11 sec. or more. When only a monitoring lead is available, a more accurate statement would be:

"Duration of the QRS due to a VPC is

_____ longer than

_____ shorter than

_____ equal to

the QRS duration of the supraventricular complexes."

longer than

15.

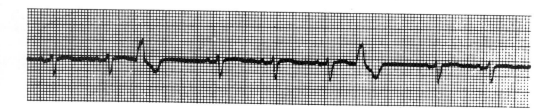

What is the QRS duration in the VPC's?

_____ sec.

0.10

What is the QRS duration in the sinus cycles?

_____ sec.

0.07

16.

A VPC DOES NOT INTERRUPT RHYTHM OF THE SINUS NODE

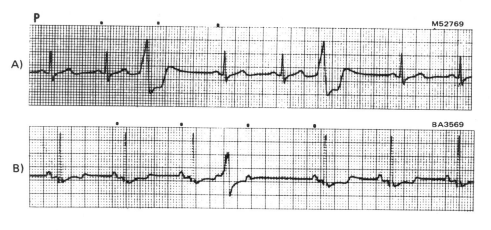

The depolarization wave causing a VPC usually does not make its way backward through the A-V junction and up into the atria. Therefore, because the VPC does not discharge the sinus node, the rhythm of the P waves continues without interruption.

17. In frame 16 what is the P-P interval?

A	B
_____ sec.	_____ sec.

A	B
0.84	*0.96*

Is the rhythm of the sinus node upset by the VPC's?

A	B
_____	_____

A	B
No	*No*

18.

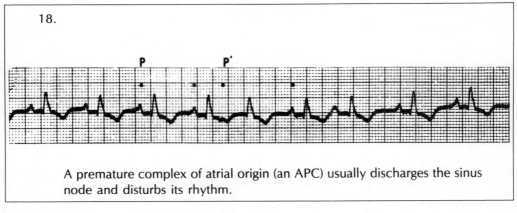

A premature complex of atrial origin (an APC) usually discharges the sinus node and disturbs its rhythm.

19. In frame 18 what is the P-P interval?

_____ sec.   *0.64*

Is the rhythm of the sinus node upset by the APC?

_____   *Yes*

20. A premature complex which does not disturb the sinus rhythm is followed by a pause which is _____.   *compensatory.*

21. The pause following a premature complex is compensatory if it is long enough to compensate for the prematurity of the early cycle.

22. **A VPC usually is followed by a compensatory pause.**

There are so many exceptions, it is wise to put little reliance in the dictum: A VPC is followed by a compensatory pause.

In reality, **following a VPC the pause may be more or less than the traditional compensatory duration.**

23.

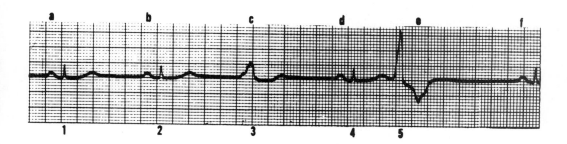

QRS No. 3 is a VPC. Does it interrupt the atrial rhythm?

_____

No. P wave d comes at the expected time.

QRS No. 5 also is a VPC. Does it interrupt the atrial rhythm?

_____

Yes. P wave f comes earlier than expected.

Why? _____

_____

_____

Retrograde conduction has occurred. P wave e is superimposed on the nadir of the T wave. This retrograde wave has depolarized (and reset) the sinus node.

RETROGRADE CONDUCTION

24. Although A-V junctional tissue does have some prejudice regarding impulses of lower origin, **unidirectional conduction** is not a hard and fast rule. Some VPC's are associated with retrograde conduction to the atria, discharge the sinus node and interrupt the rhythm of the sinus node.

25.

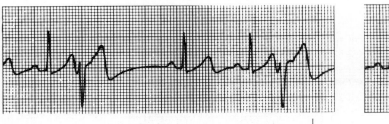

In this instance, the pause following the VPC is more than compensatory. Identify the retrograde P waves.

26. The less reliance you put on compensatory pause, the better you will like electrocardiography.

INTERPOLATED VPC'S

27. Some VPC's are followed by no pause whatsoever. The interval between the two normal cycles is adequate to squeeze in a VPC. A VPC which is squeezed in without subsequent pause is **interpolated.**

28.

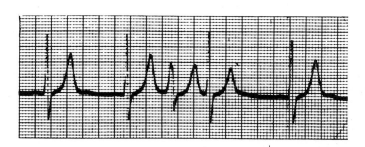

Is there a pause following this VPC?

_____   *No*

The VPC comes at just the lucky moment; the sinus beat follows without any
interruption. This VPC is described as

_____.   *interpolated.*

END-DIASTOLIC VPC

29. Occasionally a VPC may occur so late in diastole that the sinus P wave
already has put in its appearance.

30.

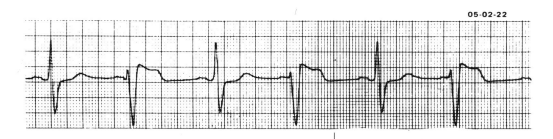

05-02-22

In the above strip, each end-diastolic
VPC is preceded by a P wave, but is it
preceded by a *premature* P wave?

_____   *No.*

31. A VPC apparently is dependent upon the preceding impulse. Fixed coupling describes the constant interval which usually separates VPC's from their antecedent cycles.

32.

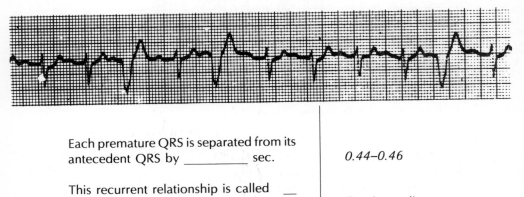

Each premature QRS is separated from its antecedent QRS by _____ sec.

0.44–0.46

This recurrent relationship is called _____ .

fixed coupling.

33. **Fixed coupling** describes the constant interval which ordinarily separates VPC's from their antecedent cycles. **Variable coupling** alerts one to the possibility of something a little different.

34.

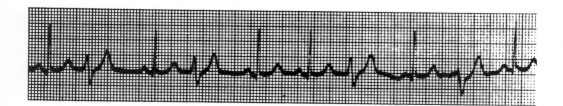

Measure the coupling intervals of the four premature complexes.

_____, _____, _____, _____sec.

What other feature is present in the cycle with an atypical coupling interval?

0.44, 0.44, 0.46, 0.56 secs.
Configuration is different from the three VPC's with fixed coupling. Also, this premature QRS is preceded by a premature P wave.

VENTRICULAR PARASYSTOLE

35. VPC's with a variable coupling interval are suggestive of **parasystole.**

This term describes the behavior of an independent ectopic focus which is protected from the dominant rhythm. The parasystolic focus becomes manifest if its discharge occurs at a time when the ventricles are not refractory. Thus, the interectopic intervals have a common denominator.

36.

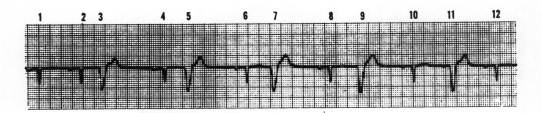

This strip illustrates ventricular parasystole. Two of the characteristics of ventricular parasystole are:

1. _____

2. _____

1. VPC's with variable coupling.

2. The interectopic intervals are constant or have a common denominator.

---

37. **Fusion beats** are a third characteristic of ventricular parasystole. This is illustrated in complex No. 11, frame 36. Note the preceding P wave. Excitation from above and excitation from the ventricular focus occurred about the same time. Each was responsible for depolarization of a portion of the ventricles. Thus, in a fusion beat, QRS presents features of both supraventricular and ectopic ventricular origin.

VPC-ON-T

38. A VPC may occur so early that it lands on the T wave of the previous cycle. A **VPC-on-T** is especially likely to trigger ventricular tachycardia or fibrillation.

However, late VPC's also may precipitate ventricular tachycardia or fibrillation.

39.

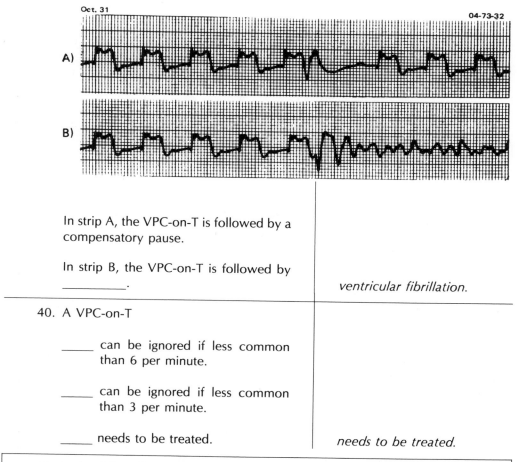

Oct. 31

04-73-32

A)

B)

In strip A, the VPC-on-T is followed by a compensatory pause.

In strip B, the VPC-on-T is followed by

_____.

ventricular fibrillation.

40. A VPC-on-T

_____ can be ignored if less common than 6 per minute.

_____ can be ignored if less common than 3 per minute.

_____ needs to be treated.

needs to be treated.

41. In the CCU, all VPC's are important but special attention is given if VPC's are:

1. Frequent.

2. Of different shapes.

3. Increasing in frequency.

4. On the T wave of the previous cycle.

5. In pairs or triplets.

42.

8:00 A.M.

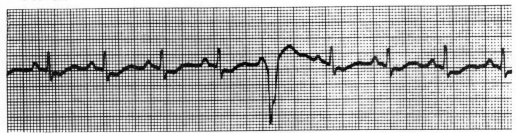

1:15 P.M.

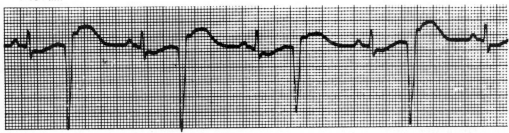

6:00 P.M.

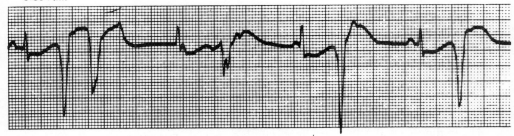

List several features which indicate that this patient's rhythm is becoming more ominous.

1. _____

2. _____

3. _____

1. VPC's are becoming more common.

2. VPC's are multiform.

3. There is a pair of VPC's.

43. **Bigeminy** refers to the occurrence of beats in groups of two. A VPC following each sinus cycle is one of the causes of bigeminy.

44.

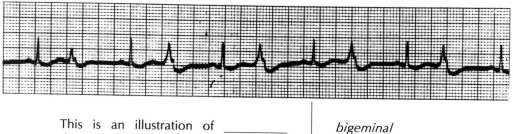

This is an illustration of _____ rhythm due to _____.

bigeminal VPC's.

45. Normal persons have occasional VPC's. These may be a nuisance but probably are not dangerous. In a person with recent myocardial infarction, VPC's are significant for two reasons:

1. They may provide warning of impending ventricular tachycardia or ventricular fibrillation.

2. Any early beat encroaches on diastole and shortens the time available for ventricular filling. Reduced filling causes reduced stroke volume.

SUMMARY—CHAPTER XIII

1. The depolarization wave causing a VPC arises within the ventricles and cannot utilize the His-Purkinje system. It is distributed slowly, via a different pathway.

2. The resultant QRS is broad and "different."

3. Usually retrograde conduction does not occur, from ventricle to atria. Therefore the rhythm of the sinus node is not disturbed by the VPC and the pause following the premature complex is compensatory.

PROBLEMS—CHAPTER XIII

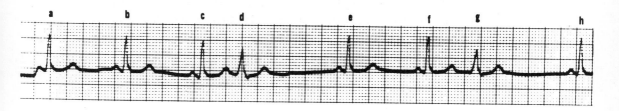

1. Describe this arrhythmia.

_____

_____

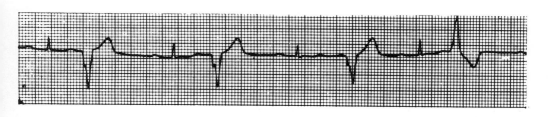

2. What are the notable features regarding these VPC's recorded during the first day after infarction?

_____

_____

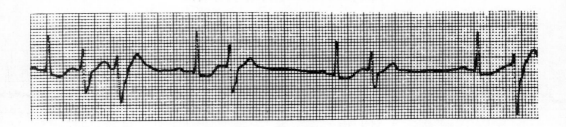

3. This rhythm strip was recorded soon after admission to the CCU. Would this patient concern you more than the patient represented in question 2?

_____

_____

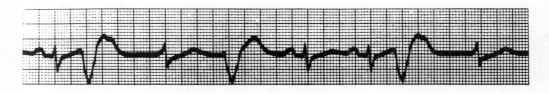

4. This rhythm strip was recorded soon after admission to the CCU. Would this patient concern you more than the patient represented in question 3?

_____

Mon. (II)

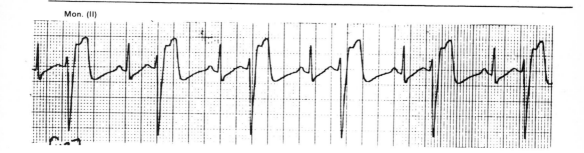

5. Describe this arrhythmia. _____

_____

Mon. (II)

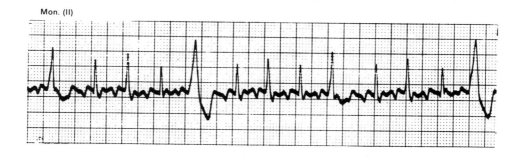

6. Describe this arrhythmia. _____

_____

chapter 14

ventricular tachycardia

1. Ventricular tachycardia consists of a series of VPC's. Thus, **two key ECG characteristics of ventricular tachycardia** already have been presented:

   1. QRS is broad and "different" from complexes of supraventricular origin.

   2. Atrial rhythm usually is undisturbed by the rhythm of the ventricles.

   Additional conventional characteristics include:

   3. Ventricular rhythm is regular or nearly regular.

   4. Rate 130–180/min.—usually.

   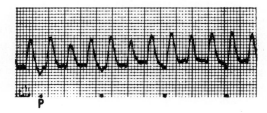

2. A depolarization wave of supraventricular origin is distributed through the ventricles via the rapidly-conducting His-Purkinje system. The resulting QRS is _____ sec. or less in the monitoring lead, unless aberrant ventricular conduction is present.

0.10

3.

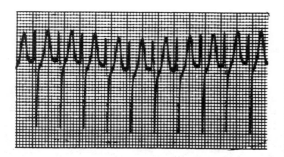

What is the QRS duration?

_____ sec.

0.07

The ectopic focus is

_____ supraventricular.

_____ ventricular.

It must be supraventricular, for QRS duration is normal. (Only impulses of supraventricular origin can make full use of the His-Purkinje rapid transit system.)

4. Supraventricular tachycardia may present abnormal and widened QRS complexes if aberrant ventricular conduction is present.

Bundle branch block and aberrant ventricular conduction produce abnormal, widened QRS complexes even though the focus driving the ventricles is in the atria or A-V junction.

5. When an ectopic beat arises in the ventricles, the QRS complex is

_____ broad (0.11 sec. or more).

_____ narrow (0.10 sec. or less).

_____ different from the sinus cycles.

_____ same as in the sinus cycles.

broad.

different from the sinus cycles.

Mon. (II)

6. Ventricular tachycardia may last for seconds, minutes or hours.

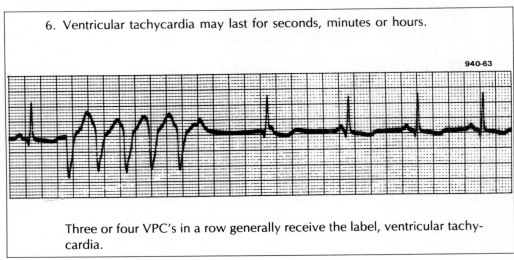

940-63

Three or four VPC's in a row generally receive the label, ventricular tachycardia.

7. QRS complexes during the bout of ventricular tachycardia shown in frame 6, are

_____ broader than in the sinus cycles.

_____ abnormal.

_____ different from the sinus cycles.

All three answers are correct.

8. A tachycardia with QRS of normal duration must be of supraventricular origin. But when dealing with a broad QRS tachycardia there always are two possibilities:

1. _____

2. _____

1. ventricular tachycardia

2. supraventricular tachycardia with aberrant ventricular conduction

---

9. Indicate the usual characteristics of ventricular tachycardia and supraventricular tachycardia.

CHARACTERISTIC	ORIGIN			*Ventricular*	*Supra-ventricular*
	Ventric-ular	Supra-ventric-ular			
QRS configuration abnormal	_____	_____		*X*	
QRS duration normal	_____	_____			*X*
QRS broad	_____	_____		*X*	
QRS configuration normal	_____	_____			*X*
QRS complexes resemble VPC's	_____	_____		*X*	

A-V DISSOCIATION

10. An ectopic impulse arising in the ventricles ordinarily is not conducted in retrograde direction through the A-V junction. Thus, ventricular tachycardia ordinarily does not disturb the rhythm of the sinus node.

    A-V dissociation is the term which describes independent, unrelated rhythms in atria and ventricles.

11.

Mon. (II)

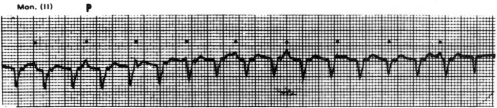

This strip shows several features of ventricular tachycardia.

Ventricular rate? _____ /min.   *168*

QRS duration? (Be sure to include the small, terminal negative wave.)
_____ sec.   *0.13*

Ventricular rhythm fairly regular?
_____   *Yes*

Atrial rate? _____ /min.   *94*

A-V dissociation (P waves unrelated to the QRS complexes)? _____   *Yes*

12.

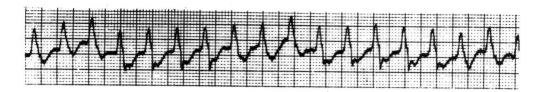

This is lead V2 from the same ECG shown in frame 11.

Are P waves seen? _____

No. This is a common problem with ventricular tachycardia. Independent P waves often are not demonstrated in any of the standard leads; small P waves easily are overshadowed by the larger QRST deflections.

---

13. Therefore, a broad QRS tachycardia with fairly regular rhythm often must be treated as if it were ventricular tachycardia, though the electrocardiographic diagnosis seldom is definite.

14.

Mon. (II)

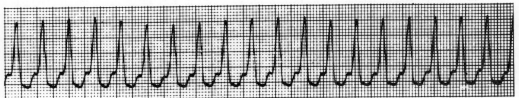

A CCU patient develops profound shock soon after the onset of this rhythm. He has received no digitalis. QRS is broader than it was during sinus rhythm and is quite different in configuration.

Standing orders call for precordial shock by the nurse if ventricular tachycardia is associated with alarming hemodynamic deterioration.

Which features of ventricular tachycardia are illustrated in this rhythm strip?

Yes   No

1. _____ _____ Fairly regular

2. _____ _____ Rate 150–200

3. _____ _____ QRS broad

4. _____ _____ Independent atrial rhythm

5. _____ _____ Fusion (Dressler) beats

What should be done. _____

_____

1. Yes

2. Yes

3. Yes

4. No

5. No.

Give precordial shock (on the basis of history and physical exam as well as ECG features).

15. An unequivocal ECG diagnosis of ventricular tachycardia seldom is possible, especially if only a monitoring lead is available.

16. Though beyond the scope of this book, history and physical examination are important in separation of ventricular tachycardia from atrial (supraventricular) tachycardia with aberrant conduction.

1. Atrial tachycardia tends to recur over a period of years. Atrial tachycardia occurs in people without heart disease and may not disturb the performance of the heart too badly. Atrial tachycardia frequently is terminated by carotid massage. Atrial tachycardia is a rare complication in the first day of myocardial infarction.

2. Ventricular tachycardia seldom causes recurrent brief spells over a period of years. Ventricular tachycardia more commonly occurs in people with heart disease and more commonly seriously decreases the performance of the heart, causing peripheral vascular collapse. Carotid sinus massage is not likely to terminate ventricular tachycardia. Ventricular tachycardia is common during the first day or two of myocardial infarction.

17. This tracing was from a young woman who walked into the emergency room complaining of the same sort of spell she had had repeatedly since childhood. Color was good. Skin was warm.

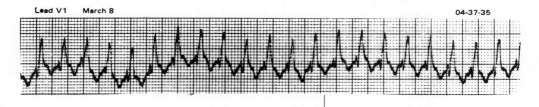

Lead V1   March 8   04-37-35

Atrial rate and rhythm _____

Ventricular rate and rhythm _____

QRS duration _____

This broad QRS tachycardia could be

_____ ventricular tachycardia.

_____ atrial tachycardia with aberrant ventricular conduction.

No P waves seen.

208/min. Regular.

0.11 sec.

either

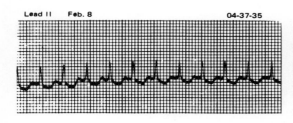

Lead II   Feb. 8   04-37-35

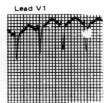

Lead V1

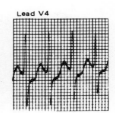

Lead V4

In her ECG folder you find this record obtained during a prior admission.

Given this history, what diagnosis is most likely for the arrhythmia of March 8?

Atrial tachycardia with aberrant ventricular conduction.

18. Although an unequivocal ECG diagnosis of ventricular tachycardia seldom is possible, a convincing conclusion is likely when certain clues are present.

    Helpful clues in making a diagnosis of ventricular tachycardia include:

    1. Prior tracings when sinus rhythm was present show different QRS configuration. (See frames 19 and 20.)

    2. The nature of "warning beats." Premature complexes which preceded onset of the tachycardia are definite VPC's. (See frames 21, 22, and 23.)

    3. Dressler or capture beats. (See frames 24, 25, 26, and 27.)

    4. Special leads show P waves uninterrupted by the ectopic ventricular rhythm. (See frames 28, 29, and 30.)

    5. The first beat of the paroxysm is identified as a definite VPC. (See frame 22.)

19. You admit a man with dyspnea and chest distress. There have been many prior hospitalizations for obstructive lung disease.

Present record, lead II

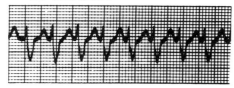

The rhythm strip shows a broad QRS tachycardia.

What could be done to decide if this is ventricular tachycardia or supraventricular tachycardia with bundle branch block?

_____

_____

Compare present QRS configuration with that during prior admissions.

20.

Old record, lead II

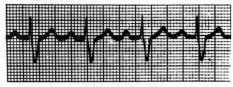

This is what you find in his ECG folder from the last admission.

What do you conclude?

_____

_____

A broad QRS complex is present even with sinus rhythm. The broad QRS tachycardia in frame 19 is supraventricular with bundle branch block.

21. The **nature of warning beats** (premature complexes during prior hours) is the clue most often helpful.

22.

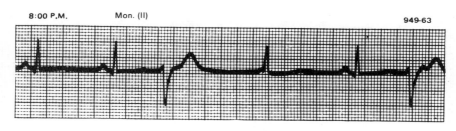

8:00 P.M.   Mon. (II)   949-63

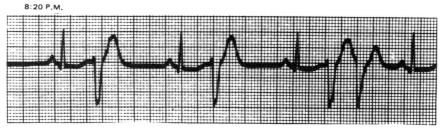

8:20 P.M.

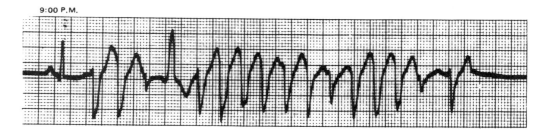

9:00 P.M.

The broad QRS tachycardia at 9:00 P.M. probably is

_____ ventricular.

_____ supraventricular with aberration.

Why?

1. _____

2. _____

3. _____

ventricular.

1. Because of the company it keeps—numerous VPC's.

2. Initial beat is a VPC.

3. Warning beats at 8:00 P.M. and 8:20 P.M. are VPC's.

23.

Mon. (II)   949-63

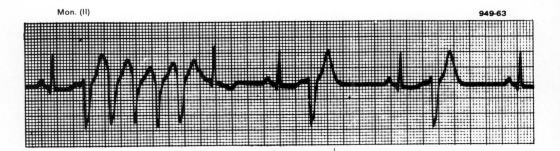

The paroxysm of broad QRS tachycardia is

_____ ventricular tachycardia.

_____ supraventricular with aberrant ventricular conduction.

What provides the clue? _____

_____

ventricular tachycardia.

There are single VPC's with similar configuration.

24.

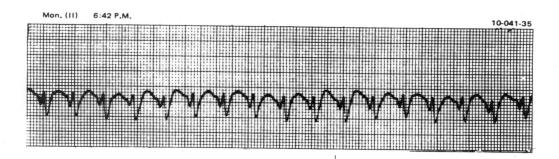

Faced with this broad QRS tachycardia and a single monitoring lead, can you make a firm diagnosis?

No.

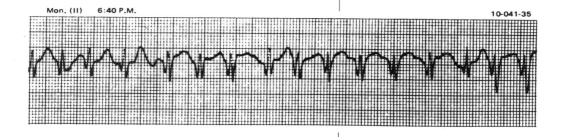

However, look at what was going on two minutes earlier! APC's were frequent. Now what do you think was going on at 6:42 P.M.?

_____

_____

Atrial tachycardia with aberrant ventricular conduction.

DRESSLER COMPLEX

25. The Dressler complex (fusion complex) is one of the most helpful clues pointing to ventricular tachycardia. In a broad QRS tachycardia, the Dressler complex is a QRS which is narrower than its associates. It comes on time or a bit early and indicates the ventricles were depolarized from two separate, nearly simultaneous impulses—one supraventricular and one from the ectopic ventricular focus.

Mon. (II)

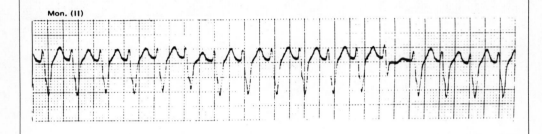

26.

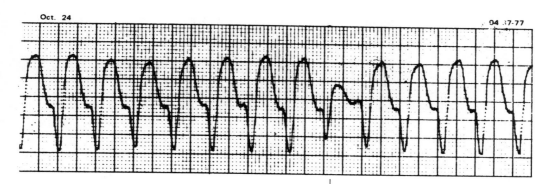

Oct. 24   04 37-77

Ventricular rate _____ /min.	*148*
QRS duration _____ /sec.	*0.10*
What is responsible for the narrow complex?	
_____	*The atria have captured the ventricles for this cycle.*
_____	

27. Unfortunately, Dressler complexes are uncommon unless the ventricular rate is below 160. If **atrial capture** (a Dressler complex) is to occur, the atrial depolarization wave must be delivered to the ventricles at just the right moment—prior to next discharge of the ectopic ventricular focus, but long enough following the preceding cycle to escape its refractory period.

28.

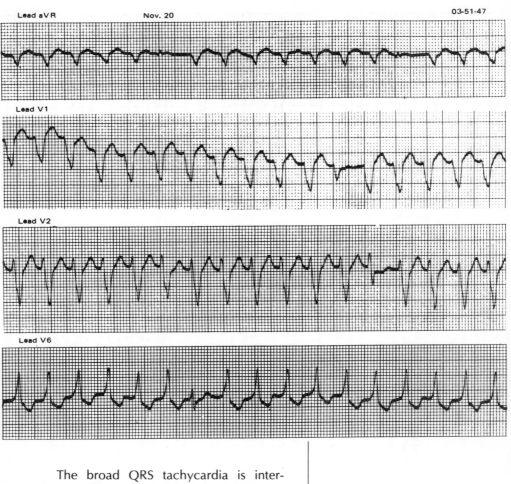

The broad QRS tachycardia is interrupted by occasional cycles which appear to be of supraventricular origin. They are _____ .

Dressler complexes.

Dressler complexes indicate that there is an independent rhythm in the _____.

atria.

29. **Independent atrial activity** often cannot be demonstrated in standard leads where small P waves are hidden by the larger QRST complexes. Special leads may show large P waves and reveal the true state of affairs, A-V dissociation.

A recording electrode within the esophagus is only a few mm. away from the left atrium. Or the tip of a pacing catheter advanced into the right atrium can be used to record an atrial electrogram.

30.

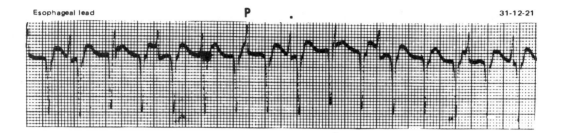

Esophageal lead   P   31-12-21

P waves are large because the esophageal electrode is close to the atria. Two of the P waves are marked. Locate the others.

What is the P-P interval? _____ sec.   *0.56 sec.*

What is the atrial rate? _____ /min.   *108/min.*

What is the R-R interval? _____ sec.   *0.38 sec.*

What is the ventricular rate?
_____ /min.   *152/min.*

What clue is provided by identification of P waves?

_____

_____

A-V dissociation present.
Atrial and ventricular activity are not related.

31.

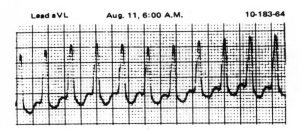

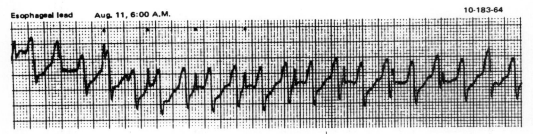

Some P waves are marked. Locate the others.

The diagnostic possibilities include:

_____ Atrial tachycardia with aberrant ventricular conduction and 2:1 A-V block.

No. Atrial rhythm is completely independent.

_____ Ventricular tachycardia with retrograde V-A conduction.

No. The R-P interval is completely variable.

_____ Ventricular tachycardia without retrograde conduction.

Yes. This is a fairly regular broad QRS tachycardia with independent atrial rhythm.

---

32. A humble approach to the broad QRS tachycardia is wise, for:

1. A changing P-QRS relationship does not prove A-V dissociation and ventricular tachycardia. It may indicate **changing retrograde V-A conduction.**

2. A constant P-QRS relationship does not exclude ventricular tachycardia. It may indicate **stable retrograde V-A conduction.**

33.

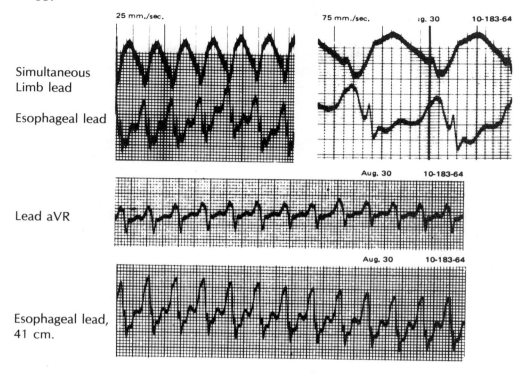

Simultaneous
Limb lead

Esophageal lead

Lead aVR

Esophageal lead,
41 cm.

These records were obtained during another episode of broad QRS tachycardia
occurring in the same patient represented in frame 31.

Which of the following statements apply?

_____ P could be the cause of QRS.

_____ QRS could be the cause of P.

_____ This could be ventricular tachycardia with retrograde V-A conduction.

_____ This could be atrial tachycardia
with aberrant ventricular conduction.

Each statement is a
correct possibility.

TREATMENT

34. A broad QRS tachycardia in a desperately sick patient often must be treated as though it were ventricular tachycardia, though the diagnosis is tentative. If lidocaine is not promptly effective, **precordial shock** is used.

35.　　　　BIDIRECTIONAL VENTRICULAR TACHYCARDIA

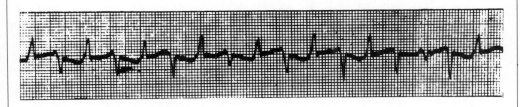

This less common form of broad QRS tachycardia is particularly suggestive of digitalis toxicity. Because the QRS complexes alternate in direction it is called **bidirectional ventricular tachycardia,** though by this point in chapter XIV, it is apparent that other diagnostic possibilities exist.

ACCELERATED IDIOVENTRICULAR RHYTHM

36. Another term must be mentioned in this chapter, with apologies for word usage.

    Accelerated idioventricular rhythm sometimes is called **slow ventricular tachycardia** or **accelerated junctional rhythm with aberrant ventricular conduction.** Because of the reasonable rate, there is not much hemodynamic upset. Prognosis is not very serious.

Mon. (II)

Continuous strip

04-70-75

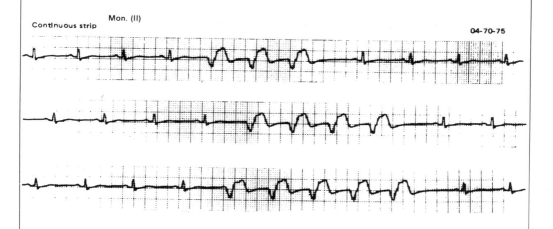

Characteristics of accelerated idioventricular rhythm include:

1. Rate usually 60–100/min.

2. Brief duration, usually less than a dozen complexes.

3. Bout of AIR usually initiated by a late diastolic VPC, or by ventricular escape in the setting of sinus slowing.

SUMMARY—CHAPTER XIV

1. Ventricular tachycardia is fairly regular, at a rate of 130–180/min.

2. The QRS complexes have features of a series of VPC's.

3. Atrial rhythm is not disturbed. The atrial and ventricular rhythms are unrelated, an example of A-V dissociation.

4. A broad QRS tachycardia may be ventricular or it could be supraventricular with aberrant ventricular conduction.

5. Helpful clues leading to a diagnosis of ventricular tachycardia include:

1. Previous VPC's of similar configuration.
2. First beat of the paroxysm is a VPC.
3. Dressler beats.

PROBLEMS—CHAPTER XIV

Continuous strip

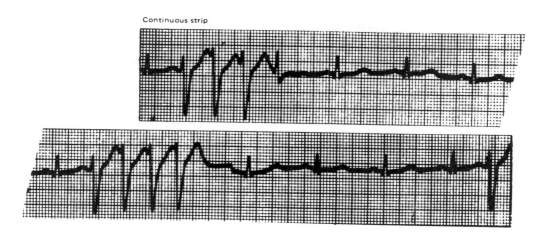

1. Spells of giddiness and palpitation were the chief complaint of this middle-aged diabetic with angina at rest during the prior three days. A 12-lead tracing was indicative of acute anterior injury. What are the bursts of tachycardia seen in this continuous strip?

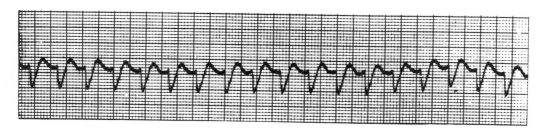

2. What is the arrhythmia?

3. If circumstances permitted, what else would you like to know to assist in making a diagnosis?

4. A) Construct a ladder diagram, assuming the atrial rate is 60/min. (P-P 1.0 sec.)

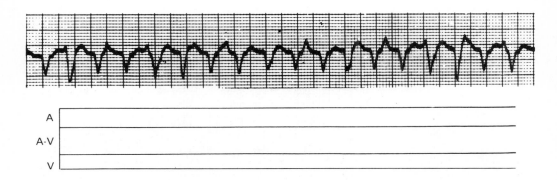

B) Construct a ladder diagram, assuming the atrial rate is 120/min. (P-P 0.5 sec.)

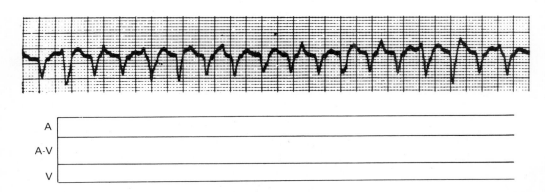

C) Using either hypothesis, the atrial and ventricular mechanisms are unrelated and the probable rhythm diagnosis is _____.

5. A) Construct a ladder diagram, assuming the atrial rate is 32/min. (P-P 1.84 sec.)

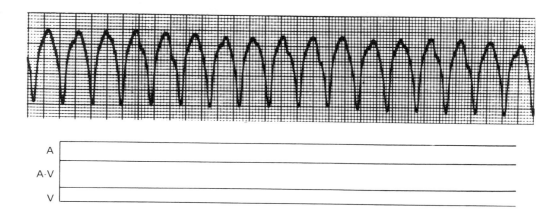

A

A-V

V

B) Construct a ladder diagram using an alternate hypothesis.

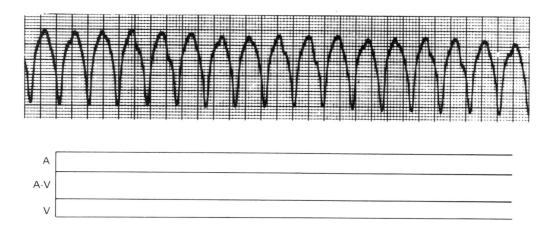

A

A-V

V

6.

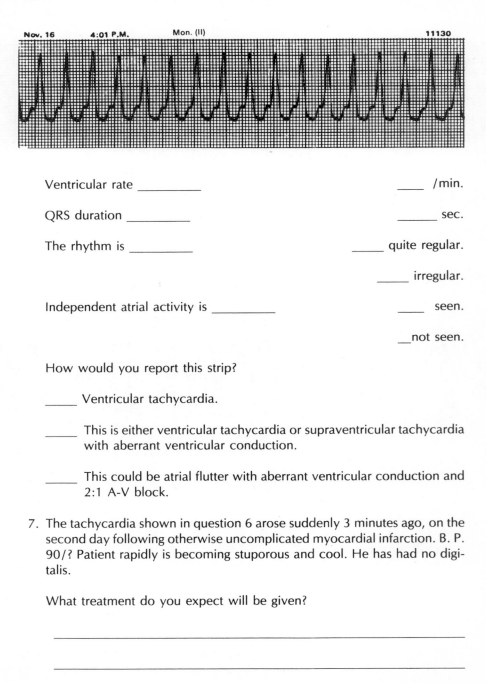

Nov. 16   4:01 P.M.   Mon. (II)   11130

Ventricular rate _____   ____ /min.

QRS duration _____   _____ sec.

The rhythm is _____   _____ quite regular.

                                           _____ irregular.

Independent atrial activity is _____   ____ seen.

                                           __not seen.

How would you report this strip?

_____ Ventricular tachycardia.

_____ This is either ventricular tachycardia or supraventricular tachycardia with aberrant ventricular conduction.

_____ This could be atrial flutter with aberrant ventricular conduction and 2:1 A-V block.

7. The tachycardia shown in question 6 arose suddenly 3 minutes ago, on the second day following otherwise uncomplicated myocardial infarction. B. P. 90/? Patient rapidly is becoming stuporous and cool. He has had no digitalis.

What treatment do you expect will be given?

_____

_____

ventricular flutter and fibrillation

1.

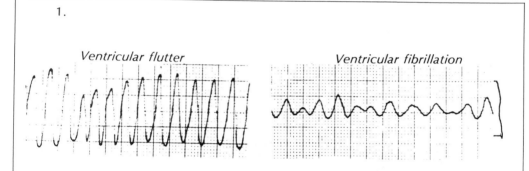

Ventricular flutter

Ventricular fibrillation

Ventricular flutter is similar to rapid ventricular tachycardia. The deflections are fairly uniform, the rhythm reasonably regular, and the rate above 220/min. However, in contrast to ventricular tachycardia there are no intervening ST segments or T waves. Ventricular flutter often progresses to ventricular fibrillation.

Ventricular fibrillation describes the chaos when a coordinated depolarization wave is replaced by a disorganized state in which groups of cells are discharged without regard to their neighbors. At any one moment, different fibers are found in different states of electrical and mechanical activity. Therefore, the QRS complex, ST segment, and T waves are absent.

Ventricular fibrillation is characterized *electrically* by irregular undulations of variable contour and amplitude without recognizable QRST complexes. Ventricular fibrillation is characterized *mechanically* by a quivering ventricle, ineffective as a pump.

2. Chaotic, irregular depolarization of the ventricles is called _____	*ventricular fibrillation.*

3. Chaotic, variable ventricular depolarization waves are present in

_____ ventricular flutter.

_____ atrial fibrillation.

_____ ventricular fibrillation.

ventricular fibrillation.

---

4. Effective circulation stops with the onset of ventricular fibrillation. It is the major cause of cardiac arrest and in the CCU usually can be reversed by precordial shock.

5.

A)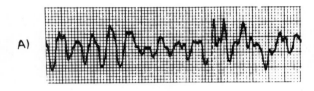

B)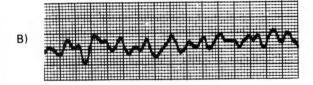

These are examples of ventricular fibrillation.

Well-defined, uniform QRS complexes are

_____ present.

_____ absent.

absent.

6. Artifact (such as a loose electrode) might cause a pattern similar to that shown in frame 5. A glance at the patient will help to distinguish artifact from ventricular fibrillation. The patient with ventricular fibrillation soon appears _____.

lifeless.

TREATMENT

7. Distinction between ventricular flutter and fibrillation often is arbitrary and without much meaning. The clinical picture is the same—absent cardiac output. Treatment is the same—precordial shock.

8.

Mon. (II)

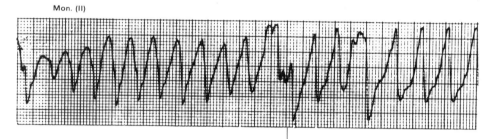

Would you call this ventricular tachycardia, ventricular flutter or ventricular fibrillation? _____

_____

Neither term fits well. The pattern is too irregular for typical tachycardia or flutter, too regular for fibrillation.

If the patient developed the above strip and promptly became lifeless, your diagnosis would be _____

_____

ventricular fibrillation or flutter.

9. These strips were recorded at intervals of about 30 seconds. The patient lost consciousness by the time strip D was recorded. The artifact of precordial shock appears midway through strip D.

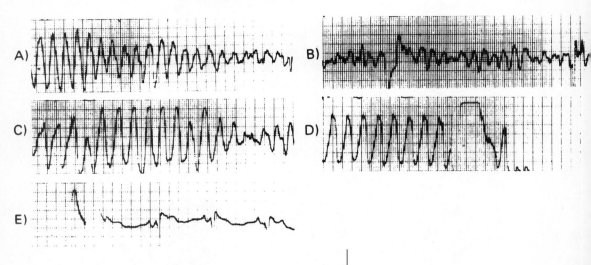

These strips illustrate:

True	False		
_____	_____	Ventricular flutter may change to fibrillation.	*True. (Note strip A.)*
_____	_____	Ventricular fibrillation may change to flutter.	*True. (Note change from strip B to C)*
_____	_____	Distinguishing between ventricular flutter and fibrillation usually is an academic exercise of little clinical value.	*True.*
_____	_____	Ventricular fibrillation is incurable.	*False. (Note sinus rhythm in strip E.)*

10. Though ventricular fibrillation may develop without warning, preceding ventricular tachycardia or VPC's commonly are seen.

11.

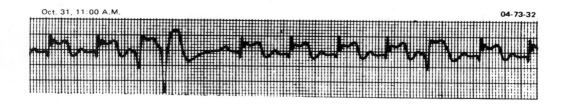

Oct. 31, 11:00 A.M.   04-73-32

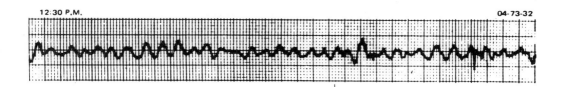

12:30 P.M.   04-73-32

What is the rhythm at 12:30 P.M.?	*Ventricular fibrillation*
At 11:00 A.M. what warned of the high risk of ventricular fibrillation?	*VPC-on-T.*
	VPC's in pairs.
	Multiform configuration of the VPC's may be important.
	Pronounced ST elevation suggests that the injury is acute. (During early hours of infarction, VPC's are more ominous than those during convalescence.)

12. Although a totally disorganized pattern is the rule, some patients with ventricular fibrillation do have a recurrent wave simulating QRS.

In a setting of sudden death, this would not deter treatment—precordial shock.

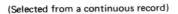

(Selected from a continuous record)

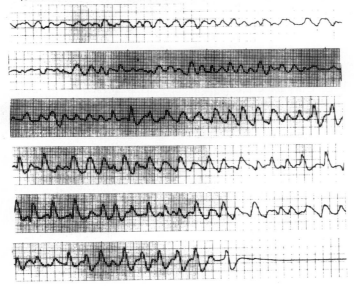

13. When the clinical picture is that of sudden death, but the ECG does not show the classic chaotic pattern of ventricular fibrillation

_____ try precordial shock.

_____ wait for the classic picture to appear.

try precordial shock.

14. The artifact of chest compression (external cardiac massage) occurs at a rate determined by the rate of chest compression. Configuration of the artifact is unpredictable.

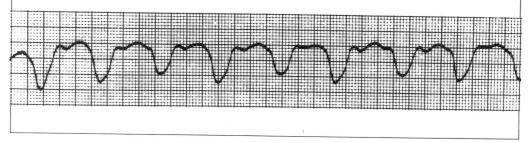

15.

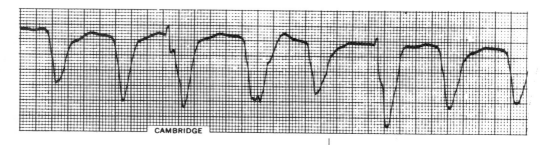

This represents

_____ a wide, bizarre QRS.

_____ chest compression artifact.

chest compression artifact.

SUMMARY—CHAPTER XV

1. During ventricular fibrillation there are irregular undulations without recognizable QRS complexes.

2. Cardiac output stops, followed by syncope and death.

3. Precordial shock is the only generally effective treatment.

4. Ventricular flutter presents uniform deflections at a very fast rate, without intervening isoelectric baseline. Clinical significance and treatment are similar to fibrillation.

PROBLEMS—CHAPTER XV

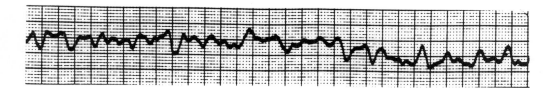

1. This is the classic pattern of _____ .

   However, it is the combination of clinical and ECG features which usually makes the diagnosis. The combination of a totally disorganized ECG pattern plus lifelessness characterize _____ .

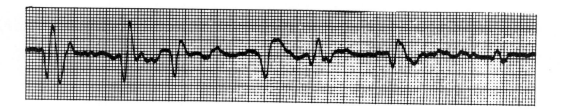

2. Although the above record does not resemble the classic fibrillation pattern shown in question 1, it if were associated with sudden lifelessness, probably it also should be treated with _____ .

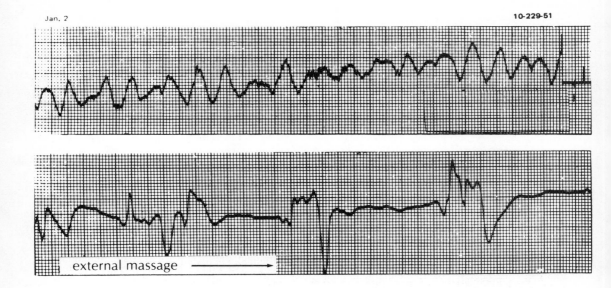

3. The top strip shows a classic pattern of ventricular fibrillation. The artifact of precordial shock is shown toward the right end. Apparently an effective beat did not resume immediately for the second strip shows a fairly flat baseline with the artifact of _____.

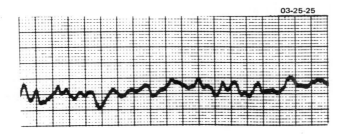

4. The patient suddenly appeared lifeless. The diagnosis is _____ .

5. The treatment is _____ .

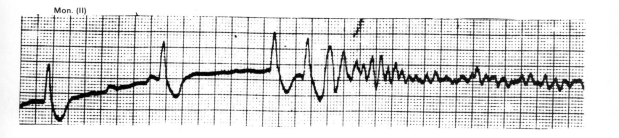

Mon. (II)

6. Describe this arrhythmia. _____

_____

chapter 16

a-v block

TERMINOLOGY

1. The word block refers to impaired conduction in the sino-atrial, junctional or His-Purkinje system.

   Traditionally, atrio-ventricular conduction is described by P-QRS relationships. However, as we shall see, the His-Purkinje system is very much involved in atrioventricular conduction. Thus, QRS configuration as well as PR interval must be considered.

   In **first degree A-V block** each P wave is conducted, but the PR interval exceeds 0.20 seconds.

   In **second degree A-V block,** some of the P waves are not conducted to the ventricles. There are two varieties. The PR interval may be either normal or long, variable or constant.

   Type I (Mobitz I or Wenckebach) second degree block describes progressive lengthening of the PR interval until one P wave is not conducted, after which the cyclic pattern is repeated. The PR interval shortens in the cycle after the pause.

   Most important, intraventricular conduction usually is normal; QRS is not broadened.

   Type II (Mobitz II) second degree A-V block is characterized by a constant PR interval, but some P waves are not conducted. The PR in the conducted cycles may be normal or prolonged.

   Most important, intraventricular conduction usually is abnormal; the broadened QRS associated with Type II second degree A-V block provides the clue that the problem is in the ventricular conduction system.

   In **third degree A-V block** none of the atrial impulses reach the ventricles. The atrial and ventricular rhythms are unrelated. Thus, the P-QRS relationship is completely variable. Generally the ventricular rhythm is regular and slow.

   High degree A-V block. Since long recordings in apparent third degree A-V block may show that an occasional P wave is conducted, it may be necessary to use this additional term. Use of this phrase is another way of saying almost complete A-V block.

FIRST DEGREE BLOCK

2. In first degree A-V block, the PR interval exceeds 0.20 seconds but each P wave is conducted.

3.

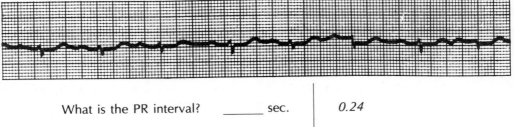

What is the PR interval? _____ sec.	*0.24*
Is each P wave conducted to the ventricles? _____	*Yes.*
This is an example of sinus arrhythmia with _____ degree A-V block.	*first*

4.

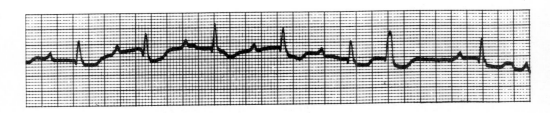

Both criteria of first degree A-V block are shown in this record.

1. Each P wave is conducted.

2. The PR interval exceeds _____ sec.

0.20 sec. (In addition there is a VPC.)

5. The major difficulty in recognizing first degree A-V block occurs when the rate is so fast or the PR so prolonged that P is hidden in the prior T wave.

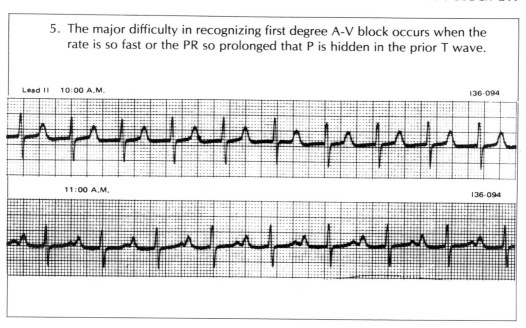

Lead II   10:00 A.M.   136-094

11:00 A.M.   136-094

6.

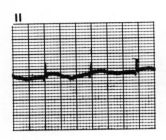
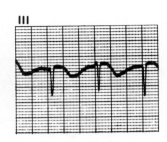
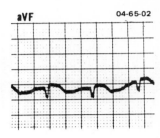

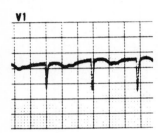
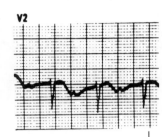
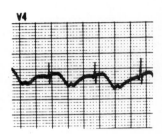

04-65-02

The P wave is not seen in leads _____ .   *II, III, aVF*

P is shown in leads _____ .   *V1, V2, V4*

The PR interval is _____ sec.   *0.30 sec.*

This is an example of _____ degree
A-V block.   *first*

SECOND DEGREE BLOCK

7. In second degree A-V block, some of the P waves are not conducted to the
ventricles. The PR interval may be either normal or prolonged, variable or
constant.

Presence or absence of QRS widening is one of the most important consid-
erations.

---

8. In second degree A-V block some P
waves are not followed by a _____
_____ .   *QRS complex.*

9. In second degee A-V block, the atrial rate is more rapid than the ventricular rate. The relationship between these rates can be described as a ratio.

10.

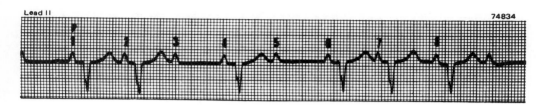

Lead II   74834

The atrial rhythm is _____.   *regular.*

The A-V ratio is _____.   *variable.*

Which P waves are conducted?
_____   *1, 2, 4, 6, 7, 8*

Which P waves are not conducted?
_____   *3, 5*

This is

_____ first degree

_____ second degree

_____ third degree   *second degree*

A-V block.

11.

Mon. (II)

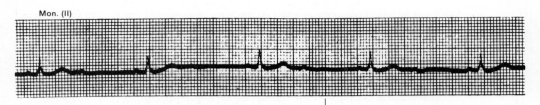

What is the atrial rate? _____ /min.	*88*
What is the ventricular rate? _____ /min.	*44*
What proportion of the atrial impulses reach the ventricles? _____	*one-half*
What is the A-V ratio? _____	*2:1*
What is the rhythm? _____	*sinus with second degree A-V block and a 2:1 ratio.*

WENCKEBACH SECOND DEGREE BLOCK

12. There are two varieties of second degree A-V block.

    Type I second degree A-V block is characterized by progressive lengthening of the PR interval until one P is not conducted, after which the cyclic pattern is repeated. The PR shortens in the cycle after the pause.

    This is the Wenckebach phenomenon.

    QRS duration usually is normal.

Mon. (II)

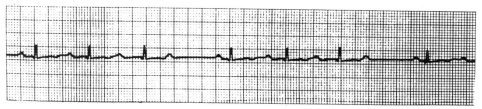

    Note progressive lengthening of PR in cycles 1–3, then the non-conducted P, the pause and finally the shorter PR.

13.

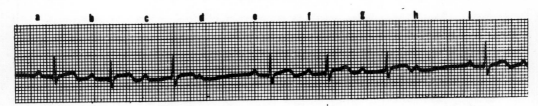

Study this tracing with special attention to the PR intervals, the P-P intervals and the R-R intervals.

The atrial rhythm is

_____ regular.

_____ irregular.

regular.

The ventricular rhythm is

_____ regular.

_____ irregular.

irregular.

The PR intervals measure:

a	b	c	d

e	f	g	h

i

0.22	*0.26*	*0.36*	*blocked*
a	*b*	*c*	*d*

0.19	*0.24*	*0.30*	*blocked*
e	*f*	*g*	*h*

0.20
i

The PR interval becomes longer with each cycle until a P wave is not followed by a QRS.

In the cycle after the non-conducted P wave, the PR interval is relatively

_____ long.

_____ short.   *short.*

This is an example of type 1 second degree A-V block, the _____ phenomenon.

Wenckebach

---

14. ECG characteristics of type 1, second degree (Wenckebach) A-V block include the following:

   _____

   _____   *PR progressively*
                                             lengthens

   _____

   _____   *A P wave periodically is*
                                             not conducted.

   _____   *PR shortens in the cycle*
                                             after the nonconducted
   _____   *P wave.*

GROUP BEATS

15. Group beats always should raise a suspicion of the Wenckebach phenomenon.

---

16. Type I (Wenckebach) second degree A-V block is not as ominous as type II:

   1. Complete block does not occur so commonly without warning.

   2. The QRS seldom is broad. The conduction disorder is not likely to involve the bundle branches.

   3. The ventricular rate does not often drop as low as may occur with type II block (see frames 18 and 20).

   4. Escape beats are not as common. When they do appear, usually they are of junctional origin (indicated by their normal QRS configuration).

TYPE II SECOND DEGREE BLOCK (MOBITZ II)

17. Now we proceed with a presentation of the other variety of second degree A-V block.

Type II second degree A-V block is illustrated below. The PR interval is constant but some P waves are not conducted. In the conducted cycles, PR may be normal or prolonged. There may be a regular ratio between P waves and QRS complexes as in Strip A. Or at irregular intervals, some P waves are not conducted as in Strips B and C below. This also is illustrated in frames 10, 18, and 20.

Most important, QRS usually is broad.

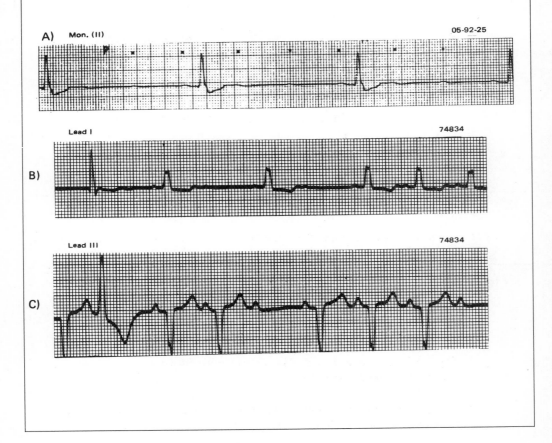

18.

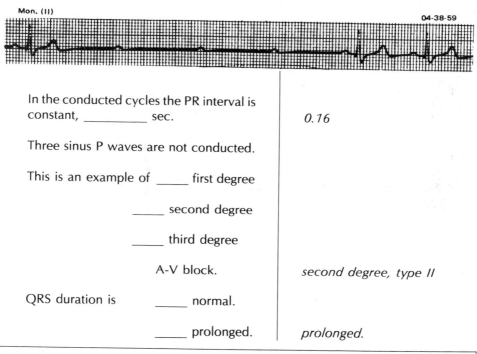

Mon. (II)   04-38-59

In the conducted cycles the PR interval is
constant, _____ sec.   *0.16*

Three sinus P waves are not conducted.

This is an example of _____ first degree

_____ second degree

_____ third degree

A-V block.   *second degree, type II*

QRS duration is   _____ normal.

_____ prolonged.   *prolonged.*

---

19. Type II second degree A-V block is an important arrhythmia following
myocardial infarction. As illustrated in frames 18 and 20, QRS often is
prolonged or slurred, indicating that the site of block is intraventricular
rather than junctional.

If type II second degree A-V block progresses, ventricular standstill may
develop with little warning.

Escape of a lower focus is necessary to prevent death. If the site of block
is intraventricular, the escape focus must be still lower in the ventricles.

Lower escape foci are slower and less reliable than those arising in junctional tissue.

20.

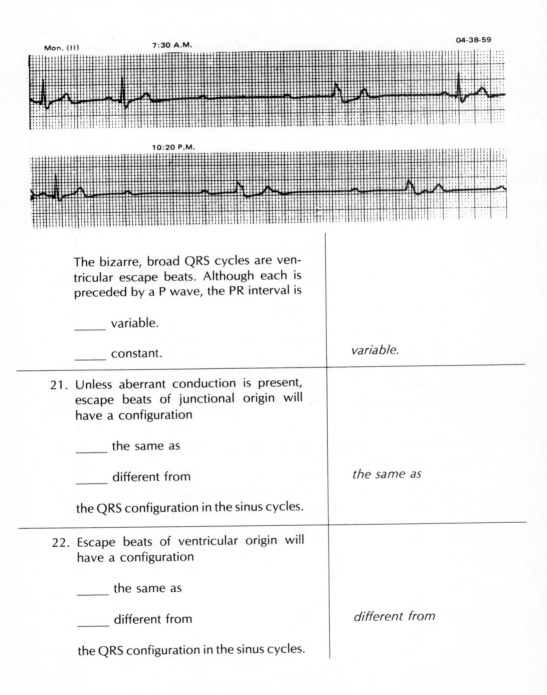

The bizarre, broad QRS cycles are ventricular escape beats. Although each is preceded by a P wave, the PR interval is

_____ variable.

_____ constant.   *variable.*

---

21. Unless aberrant conduction is present, escape beats of junctional origin will have a configuration

_____ the same as

_____ different from   *the same as*

the QRS configuration in the sinus cycles.

---

22. Escape beats of ventricular origin will have a configuration

_____ the same as

_____ different from   *different from*

the QRS configuration in the sinus cycles.

23. Escape beats are preceded by an R-R interval which is

_____ longer than

_____ shorter than   *longer than*

the standard R-R interval.

---

24. Characteristics of type II second degree A-V block may be summarized as follows:

    1. Some P waves are not conducted.

    2. In the conducted cycles the PR interval is constant.

    3. Escape beats may be seen.

    4. QRS usually is broad, reflecting damage in one of the bundle branches.

    5. Especially when QRS is broad, type II second degree A-V block warns of the development of higher degree block. Third degree A-V block will occur if both bundles become damaged.

THIRD DEGREE BLOCK

25. In third degree A-V block, none of the atrial impulses reach the ventricles. The atrial and ventricular rhythms are unrelated. The PR intervals are variable. Another term is complete heart block.

    High degree A-V block describes the situation in which the atrial and ventricular rhythms seem unrelated but in a long enough recording, a conducted P wave is found. A-V block is not quite complete.

---

26. In third degree A-V block

    _____ ⅓

    _____ none

    _____ few   *none*

    of the atrial impulses are conducted to the ventricles.

27. Therefore, in third degree block, ventricular standstill will result unless an ectopic focus develops below the block.

Escape of a junctional or ventricular pacing focus in complete A-V block is a manifestation of the inherent rhythmicity of many conduction fibers.

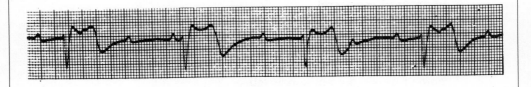

28. When a junctional ectopic cycle occurs, QRS duration is normal.

In complete heart block, if the escape focus is in the junctional tissue, the QRS duration will be

_____ normal

_____ prolonged   *normal*

unless aberrant ventricular conduction is present.

29. In complete heart block, if the ectopic pacemaker is in the ventricles, QRS configuration is _____.   *wide and "different."*

30. In third degree block, if an ectopic focus below the block does not become active, _____ will result.   *ventricular standstill*

IDIOVENTRICULAR RHYTHM

31. A slow, regular rhythm arising from a focus within the ventricles is called an idioventricular rhythm.

32. When an idioventricular rhythm is present, the ventricular pacemaker is located in the

    _____ A-V node.

    _____ sinus node.

    _____ ventricle.

ventricle.

33. The potential for automatic rhythmicity exists in many parts of the heart.

    The usual rate of discharge of the SA node is about 60–100 per minute. The usual rate of discharge of the A-V junction is about 40–60 per minute. The usual rate of discharge of an ectopic ventricular focus is about 20–40 per minute.

    If the SA node is discharging normally, and if the sinus impulses are conducted to the ventricles, the lower potential pacemakers do not have a chance to become active. They are suppressed by the higher, faster pacemaker. If the sinus node fails to discharge or if its impulse is not conducted, a lower focus may escape. The escape focus may produce a single beat or become the new, dominant pacemaker.

34. Thus some ectopic beats are not signs of "irritability" nor are they necessarily "bad." They may be evidence of the life-saving, inherent rhythmicity of the heart. They are escape beats which become manifest when the SA node does not operate or when conduction to the ventricles is blocked.

Continuous strip   During carotid sinus massage

04-78-25

35.

Mon. (II)

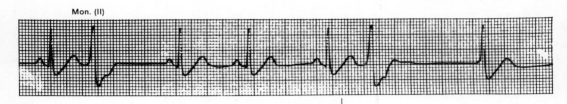

Atrial rhythm is slightly irregular, due to sinus arrhythmia.

The first VPC is followed by a compensatory pause which is terminated by a sinus cycle.

The pause following the second VPC is terminated by a _____ complex.

junctional escape

36.

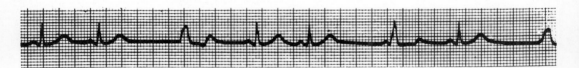

After two sinus cycles, failure of a sinus discharge permits a lower focus to _____.

escape.

The third QRS complex is broad and "different," indicating _____ origin.

ventricular

37.

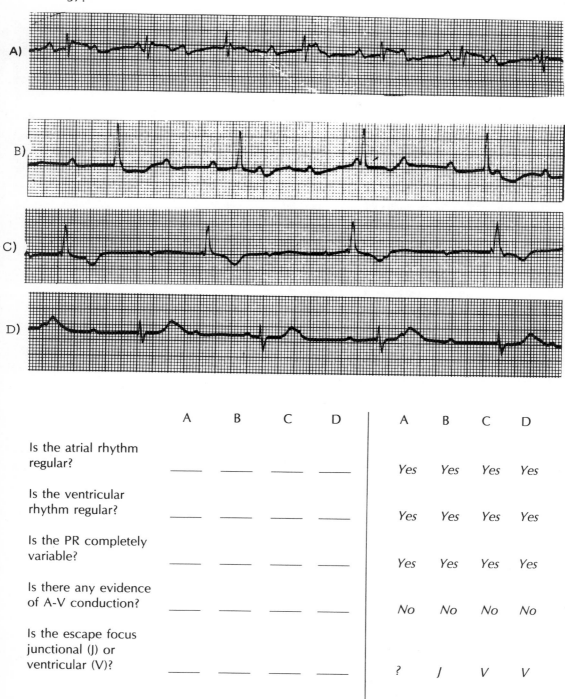

	A	B	C	D		A	B	C	D
Is the atrial rhythm regular?	___	___	___	___		Yes	Yes	Yes	Yes
Is the ventricular rhythm regular?	___	___	___	___		Yes	Yes	Yes	Yes
Is the PR completely variable?	___	___	___	___		Yes	Yes	Yes	Yes
Is there any evidence of A-V conduction?	___	___	___	___		No	No	No	No
Is the escape focus junctional (J) or ventricular (V)?	___	___	___	___		?	J	V	V

38.

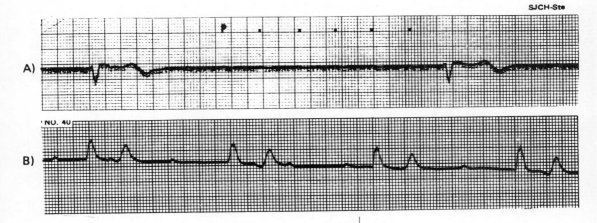

SJCH-St●

A)

'NO. 40

B)

Clinical condition in complete A-V block depends chiefly upon the stroke volume. Patient (A) was warm and awake despite ventricular rate of _____ /min. Patient (B) was cold, confused and oliguric with a rate of _____ /min.

A 13/min.

B 66/min.

---

39. In complete A-V block, the atrial mechanism may be sinus, atrial flutter or atrial fibrillation.

40.

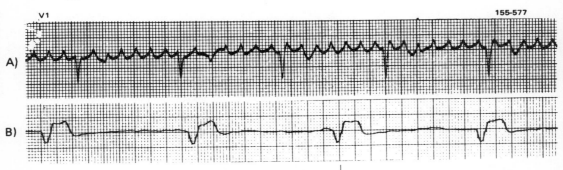

V1   155-577

A)

B)

A) Ventricular rhythm is regular and the f-R relationship varies. The atrial mechanism is _____.

flutter.

B) Ventricular rhythm is regular and the atrial mechanism is _____.

fibrillation.

41.

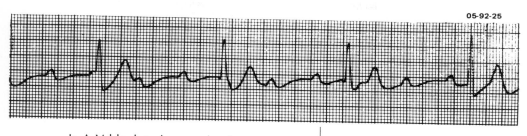

05-92-25

Is A-V block truly complete? _____

_____

No. The last QRS is narrower; probably it is a conducted or fusion complex.

Standard terminology labels this high degree A-V block, midway between second and third degree.

STOKES-ADAMS ATTACKS

42. In the presence of complete A-V block, if a reliable junctional or ventricular pacemaker does not develop, the patient may have difficulty because of an excessively slow ventricular rate.

The Stokes-Adams syndrome refers to intermittent loss of consciousness due to bradycardia or ventricular tachycardia or fibrillation accompanying complete heart block.

43.

10-229-51

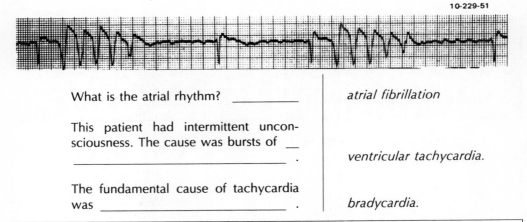

What is the atrial rhythm? _____   *atrial fibrillation*

This patient had intermittent uncon-
sciousness. The cause was bursts of __
_____ .   *ventricular tachycardia.*

The fundamental cause of tachycardia
was _____ .   *bradycardia.*

BRADYCARDIA-TACHYCARDIA

44. When bradycardia causes low cardiac output, the brain, kidneys, and heart
give signs of inadequate perfusion. Cardiac signs of inadequate perfusion
include development of various ectopic tachycardias.

Tachycardia may be a response to bradycardia.

45. An artificial pacemaker is a method of managing bradycardia or unreliable conduction.

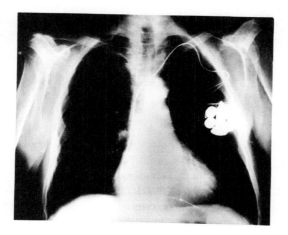

46.

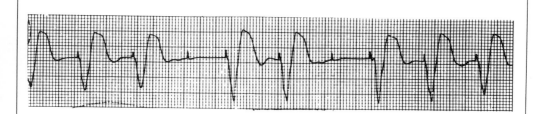

Note the blip or spike which is the electrical impulse released by the pulse generator and conducted by a pacing catheter to the cavity of the right ventricle. In this case, some spikes are not followed by a QRS; there is incomplete capture.

47. There are many types of artificial pacemakers.

A fixed-rate artificial pacemaker continues to discharge regardless of conducted beats or ectopic ventricular beats.

48.

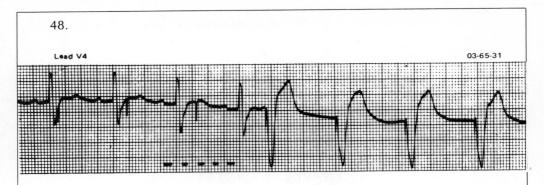

A fixed rate pulse generator and the sinus node compete for control of the ventricles. If a stimulus should occur at about the time of the apex of the T wave, there is some risk of ventricular tachycardia or fibrillation. The apex of T is considered the vulnerable period.

49. A demand pacemaker is suppressed by the appearance of a QRS, either conducted or ectopic.

If a demand pacemaker is operating properly, it will not discharge unless the asystolic interval exceeds a pre-set value. Thus, a pacing spike should not be released during the T wave, the vulnerable period.

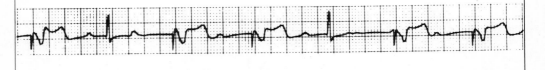

50.

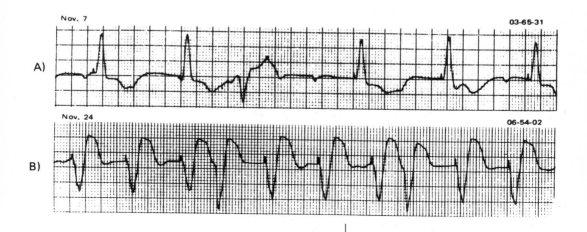

Both pacemaker patients have VPC's.
Which patient has a ventricular-inhibited
(demand) system? _____ *B*

The demand pulse generator discharges
if the asystolic interval exceeds

_____ sec. *0.68*

51.

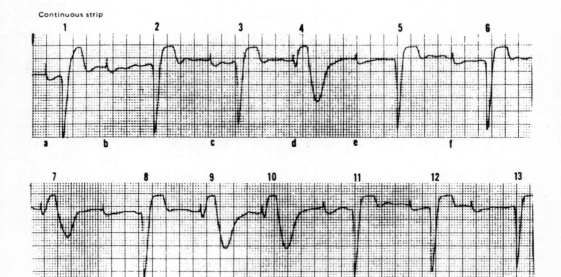

Continuous strip

A ventricular-inhibited demand pacemaker is present. Is the pacer discharge regular? _____

No.

Stimulus should occur if the asystolic interval exceeds _____ sec.

0.90 (See intervals 1-b, 2-c, 3-d, 4-e, 5-f, 7-h, 8-i, 9-j, 10-k, 11-l, and 12-m.)

Is discharge always inhibited by QRS? _____

No. QRS complexes 1 and 12 do not suppress the pulse generator.

Does each pacer spike produce a ventricular response? _____

No. There is no capture by spikes a, b, c, e, f, h, k, l, and m.

52. Although first degree, second degree, and third degree block are key terms, other aspects of A-V conduction disturbance also must be considered.

PHYSIOLOGIC A-V BLOCK

53. A-V conduction is slow or impossible for a time after passage of an excitation wave. This time is the refractory period.

If impaired conduction is due to arrival of an impulse during the refractory period, A-V block is physiologic.

54.

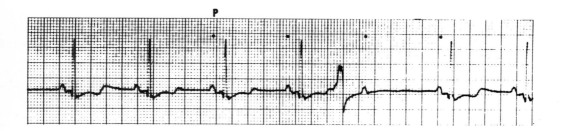

P

Why is there block of the sinus P which follows the VPC?

_____

_____

The VPC must have penetrated part of the A-V conduction system, now refractory when the sinus P arrives. This is expected A-V block.

55.

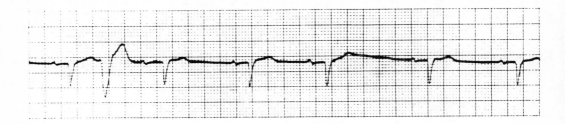

Why is the PR interval prolonged following the interpolated VPC?

_____

_____

_____

The VPC penetrated upward into the A-V conduction tissue but was blocked before discharging the atria (concealed retrograde conduction). Such recent use of the A-V junctional tissue results in slowed conduction of the subsequent sinus P wave.

56. Physiologic or expected A-V delay commonly is demonstrated by APC's.

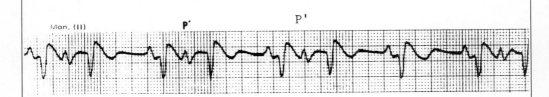

The premature P eventually is conducted to the ventricles, but with a longer PR than during the sinus cycles.

57. Atrial fibrillation always is associated with block of many of the atrial impulses.

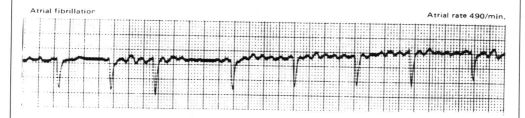

Atrial fibrillation   Atrial rate 490/min.

Atrial flutter likewise usually is associated with physiologic A-V block.

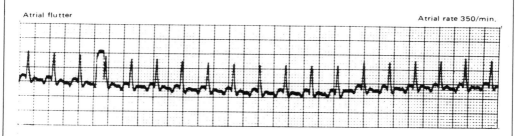

Atrial flutter   Atrial rate 350/min.

In atrial fibrillation and atrial flutter, physiologic block in the A-V junctional tissue protects the ventricles from an excessive rate of bombardment.

DIGITALIS AND A-V BLOCK

58. Digitalis is used in atrial fibrillation and flutter to prolong the refractory period in the A-V node and thereby decrease the number of atrial impulses conducted to the ventricles. Digitalis produces beneficial A-V block.

59.

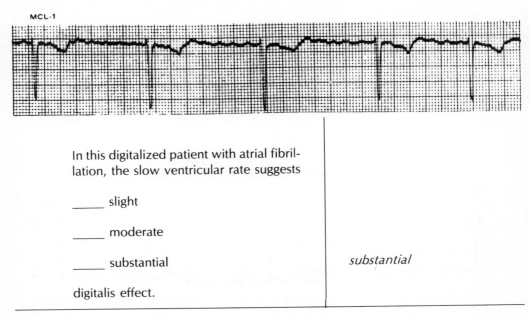

In this digitalized patient with atrial fibrillation, the slow ventricular rate suggests

_____ slight

_____ moderate

_____ substantial   *substantial*

digitalis effect.

60.

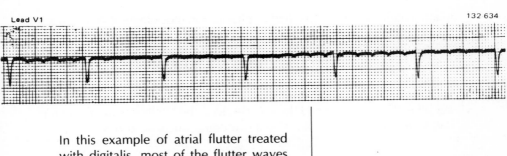

In this example of atrial flutter treated
with digitalis, most of the flutter waves
are

_____ blocked within

_____ conducted by   *blocked within*

the junctional tissue.

61. Atrial tachycardia may occur with or without A-V block.

62.

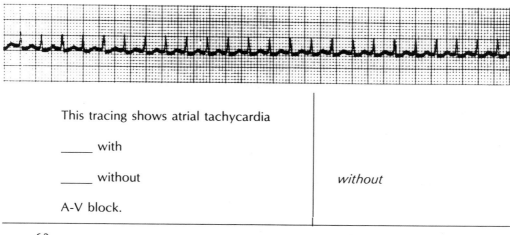

This tracing shows atrial tachycardia

_____ with

_____ without

A-V block.

without

63.

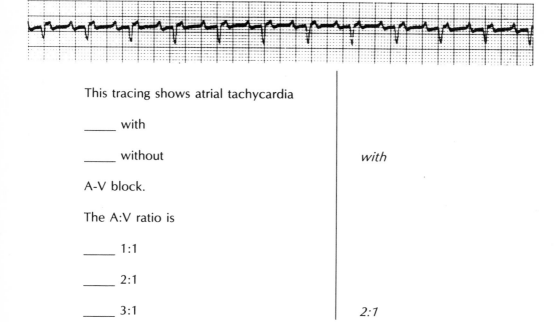

This tracing shows atrial tachycardia

_____ with

_____ without

A-V block.

The A:V ratio is

_____ 1:1

_____ 2:1

_____ 3:1

with

2:1

64. Carotid sinus massage is used to produce temporary increase in the refractory period of the A-V node. This enhances A-V block and may reveal atrial waves more clearly.

65.

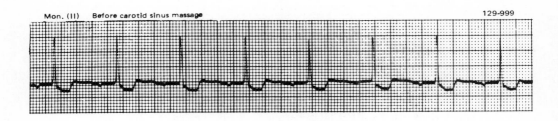

Mon. (II)   Before carotid sinus massage   129-999

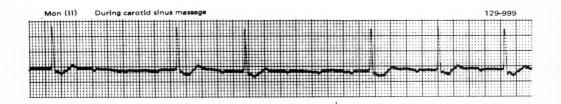

Mon (II)   During carotid sinus massage   129-999

By separating the QRS complexes, carotid sinus massage unmasks the P waves. It reveals that the atrial rate is _____ /min.

150/min.

66.

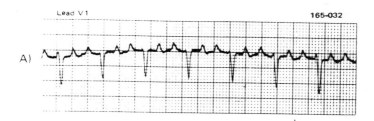

The atrial mechanism is _____ with a rate of about _____ /min. The ventricular rhythm is fairly regular at a rate of _____ /min. The A-V ratio is _____. This is an example of atrial flutter with _____ A-V conduction.

flutter
321/min.

107/min.
3:1
3:1

During carotid sinus massage.

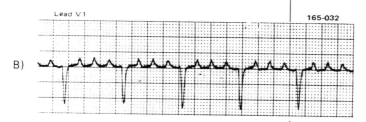

The vagal stimulation from carotid massage produced a higher degree of block. Now only

_____ ⅕

_____ ¼

_____ ⅓

¼

of the flutter waves are conducted to the ventricles.

67. Thus far, A-V block has been characterized as:

1. first degree, second degree or third degree.

2. physiologic or pathologic.

A third way of looking at A-V block is to ask about the **location** of the trouble.

SITE OF BLOCK

68. The location of atrio-ventricular block may be junctional or lower in the His-Purkinje system. If the only difficulty is **junctional,** the only manifestation will be alteration in PR interval.

If the **sub-junctional** (His-Purkinje) system is involved there will be QRS widening or some alteration of the sequence in which various areas of the ventricles are activated. QRS configuration will change, whether or not the difficulty is severe enough to cause obvious QRS broadening.

JUNCTIONAL VS. NODAL

69. The term junctional is more appropriate than nodal in most instances.

The A-V node is a discrete anatomic structure. However, new understanding causes us to use the term less frequently than before.

1. Ectopic rhythms formerly attributed to the A-V node have been demonstrated to arise from the His bundle. Indeed, the A-V node proper probably does not contain cells with the potential for automatic rhythmicity. Automatic cells *are* found in the atrio-nodal and nodal-His regions as well as the bundle itself.

2. When atrioventricular conduction is delayed, the delay often is not in the node proper but in the atrio-nodal or nodal-His region, or within one or more branches of the His bundle.

3. Furthermore, ectopic rhythms arising low in the atria cannot be distinguished from junctional beats with relatively more delay in antegrade than retrograde conduction. (See frame 54, page 122.)

70. The term junctional usually is used in place of A-V nodal to indicate an appropriate degree of vagueness regarding:

    1. the site of origin of an ectopic rhythm

    2. the site of delay in atrio-ventricular conduction.

HIS-BUNDLE RECORDS

71. New techniques permit exciting new understanding of the site of A-V delay. In the surface ECG, no deflection is produced by depolarization of the A-V node, His bundle or bundle branches. But their deflections can be recorded from intracardiac electrodes adjacent to them.

    If a pacing catheter with several electrodes is positioned with its tip in the right ventricle, proximal electrodes may lie adjacent to the right bundle, the His bundle and the atrial wall. Records from this electrode catheter might look like this sketch:

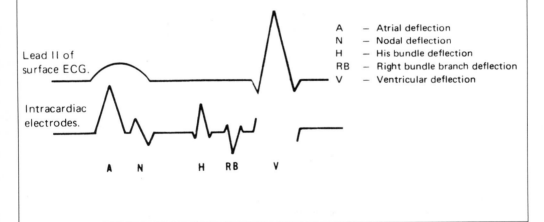

Lead II of surface ECG.

Intracardiac electrodes.

A   N   H   RB   V

A   — Atrial deflection
N   — Nodal deflection
H   — His bundle deflection
RB   — Right bundle branch deflection
V   — Ventricular deflection

72. Measuring the intervals between deflections produced by activation of various components of the junctional tissue has permitted identification of the site of block in atrio-ventricular conduction disorders.

73. From the standard ECG we can infer that location of the difficulty is junctional if only PR is altered; location is sub-junctional if duration or configuration of QRS is changed.

74.

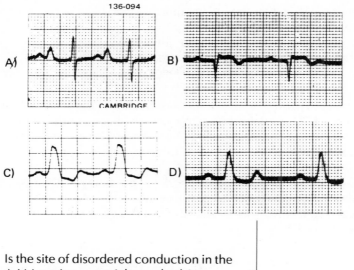

136-094

A)

CAMBRIDGE

B)

C)

D)

Is the site of disordered conduction in the A-V junction, ventricles or both?

A. _____   *A. A-V junction*

B. _____   *B. A-V junction*

C. _____   *C. Ventricles*

D. _____   *D. Both*

FASCICULAR BLOCK

75. Sub-junctional atrio-ventricular block may occur within the bundle branches or their subdivisions.

Thus, with the development of **right bundle branch block,** one of the strands upon which ventricular activation depends is not functioning.

Other strands are the anterior division of the left bundle and the posterior division of the left bundle. Disturbance here is called **divisional, fascicular** or **hemiblock.**

Or, there may be complete **left bundle branch block.**

76. If there is late activation of an entire ventricle (RBBB or LBBB), QRS is different and grossly widened.

However, if only a division of the left bundle is impaired, only the portion of the ventricle supplied by that division will be activated late.

With divisional conduction impairment (hemiblock), altered sequence of left ventricular activation may be manifest only as altered QRS configuration without notable widening.

77.

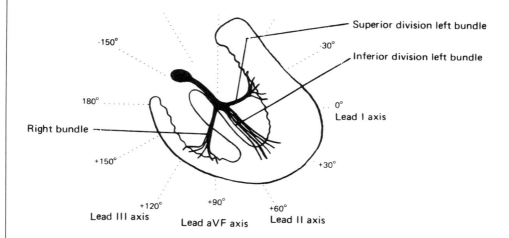

If the anterior (superior) division of the left bundle is blocked, activation will be delayed in the anterior portion of the left ventricle. The last part of QRS will represent late activation of myocardium supplied by the anterior division.

Although somewhat more is involved, superior (anterior) hemiblock is suspected when the late QRS forces are directed superiorly (headward). This is indicated by a dominant S wave in leads II, III, and aVF.

78.

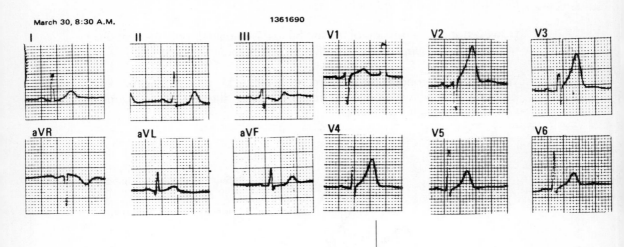

March 30, 8:30 A.M.   1361690

I   II   III   V1   V2   V3

aVR   aVL   aVF   V4   V5   V6

QRS duration is _____ sec.

0.07 sec.

The last part of QRS represents a depolarization wave moving

_____ directly away from

_____ not especially away from

not especially away from

the positive electrode in leads II and aVF (the left leg electrode).

79.

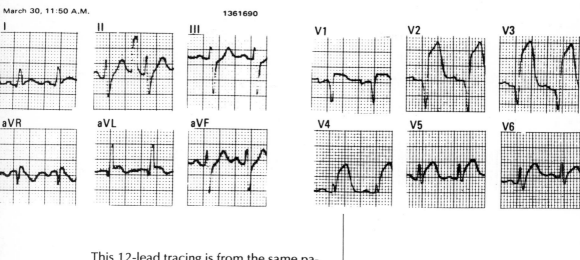

This 12-lead tracing is from the same patient represented in frame 78

In the record of 11:50 A.M., QRS duration is

_____ sec.   *about 0.08 sec.*

The terminal QRS forces are directed

_____ away from

_____ not particularly away from   *away from*

the positive electrode in leads II and aVF (left leg electrode).

Between 8:30 and 11:50 A.M., altered sequence of ventricular activation has caused substantial change in QRS configuration. This is due to left superior divisional block (left anterior hemiblock, anterior hemiblock).

80. Recognition of hemiblock indicated disturbance in one of the strands upon which atrio-ventricular conduction depends. It may warn of further trouble ahead.

81.

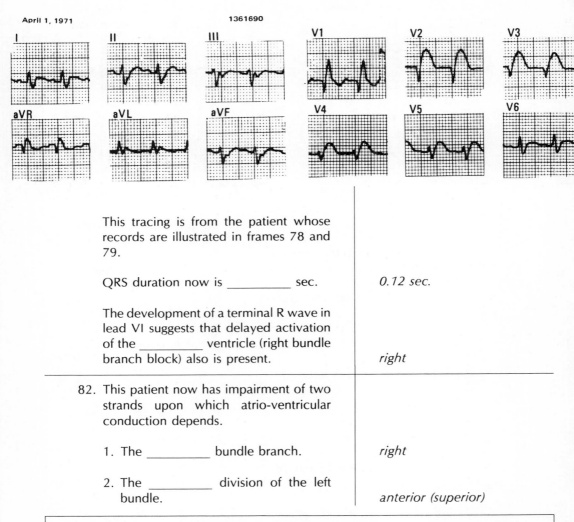

April 1, 1971   1361690

I   II   III   V1   V2   V3

aVR   aVL   aVF   V4   V5   V6

This tracing is from the patient whose
records are illustrated in frames 78 and
79.

QRS duration now is _____ sec.   *0.12 sec.*

The development of a terminal R wave in
lead VI suggests that delayed activation
of the _____ ventricle (right bundle
branch block) also is present.   *right*

82. This patient now has impairment of two
strands upon which atrio-ventricular
conduction depends.

1. The _____ bundle branch.   *right*

2. The _____ division of the left
   bundle.   *anterior (superior)*

83. The diagnosis of hemiblock may be impossible from a monitoring lead.
However, the important feature to know is that alteration in QRS duration
or configuration may indicate that the atrio-ventricular conduction apparatus is compromised.

SUMMARY—CHAPTER XVI

1. Conduction from atria to ventricles may be impaired (blocked) partially or completely. Location of the block may be in the fascicles, the bundles, or the A-V junction.

2. Some block is physiologic; thus in atrial flutter or fibrillation, many of the 300–450 impulses/min. are blocked and do not stimulate the ventricles.

3. Pathologic block in the A-V junction is considered in three grades:

   first degree: each P is conducted but the PR exceeds 0.20 sec.

   second degree:
   Type I—progressive lengthening of PR until one P is non-conducted, after which the shortest PR occurs.
   Type II—PR constant and usually normal but an occasional P is non-conducted. QRS usually prolonged or altered.

   third degree: No P waves are conducted. The ventricles are controlled by an independent focus in the A-V junction or ventricle.

PROBLEMS—CHAPTER XVI

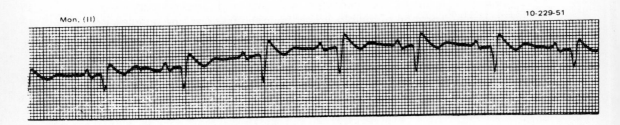

Mon. (II)   10-229-51

On the fourth day following postero-basal infarction, this 60-year-old·man had orthopnea, hypotension, and a temperature of 103 degrees. SGOT titer was 320 units.

1. Describe the rhythm strip. _____

   _____

   What is the discrepancy between the clinical findings and this ECG? __

   _____

2. His stroke volume probably is *(normal) (low)*.

3. What could you do to increase his stroke volume? _____

4. What could you do to increase his cardiac output? _____

Mon. (II)   Continuous strip   10-229-51

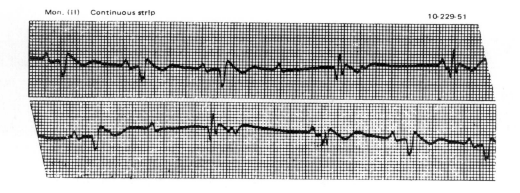

5. Later during the fourth day, the pulse slowed and became irregular. Describe this rhythm strip.

_____

_____

Mon. (II)   Continuous strip   10-229-51

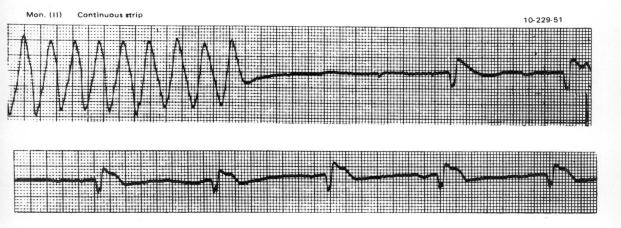

6. Still later during the fourth day, he complained of brief sinking spells. During one of them, the above record was obtained. Describe this record.

_____

_____

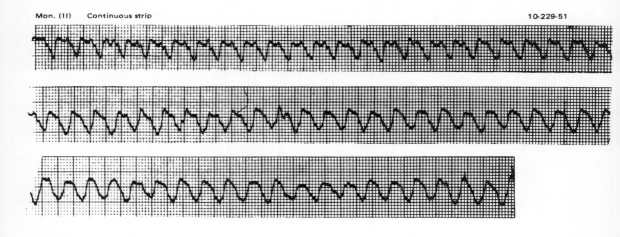

7. While his physicians were discussing matters, the above problem arose.

   Describe.

   _____

   _____

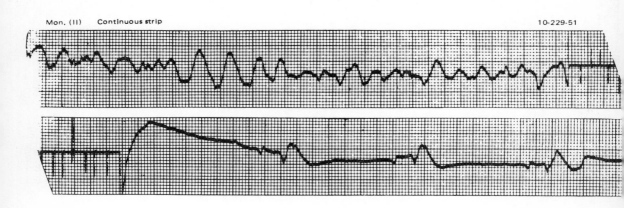

8. The patient became unconscious about this time. The nurses were active at the bedside and the above strips were recorded. Describe.

   _____

   _____

Mon., (II)   Continuous strip

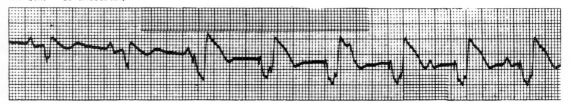

9. Finally the physicians took some definitive action. What was done?

_____

_____

Mon. (II)

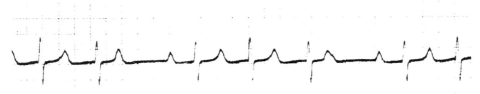

10. Describe this arrhythmia. _____

_____

This 66-year-old man was admitted at 9 P.M., April 17 with blood pressure undetectable, pulse regular at about 50/min. Portions of the 12 lead tracing are shown below. ST segment elevation in leads II, III and aVF indicate acute inferior injury.

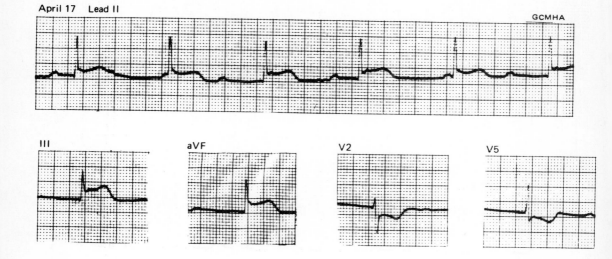

April 17   Lead II   GCMHA

III   aVF   V2   V5

11. The ventricular rhythm is *(regular) (irregular)*.

12. The atrial rhythm is *(regular) (irregular)*.

13. The PR interval is *(constant) (variable) (cyclic)*.

14. The record indicates acute inferior injury with *(1°) (2°) (3°)* A-V block.

15. The ventricles are driven by a pacemaker in the *(atria) (junctional tissue) (sub-junctional tissue)*.

16. A junctional pacemaker usually has an intrinsic rate of *(20–30/min.) (40–60/min.)*.

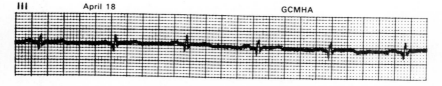

III   April 18   GCMHA

This record was obtained 24 hours later.

17. When third degree A-V block complicates acute inferior injury, the escape focus often is junctional and the A-V conduction disorder, as in this case, often is *(permanent) (transient)*.

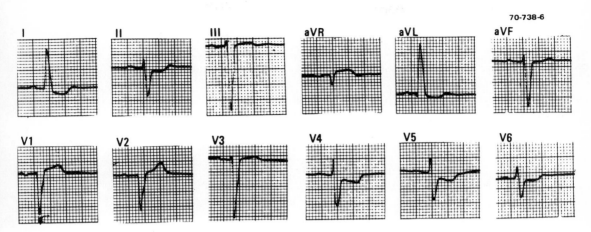

70-738-6

18. Review the lead axes, p. 273.

    In this tracing the last part of the ventricles to be depolarized is located *(superiorly and to the left) (inferiorly and to the right)*.

19. This tracing is consistent with block in the _____ division of the left bundle.

appendix

ANSWERS TO PROBLEMS—CHAPTER I

1. *sinus node*

2. *P wave*

3. *PR interval*

4. *QRS complex*

5. *broad*

ANSWERS TO PROBLEMS—CHAPTER II

1.

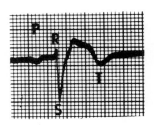 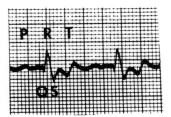

2. *the beginning of QRS.*

3. *beginning*

4.

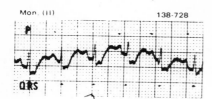

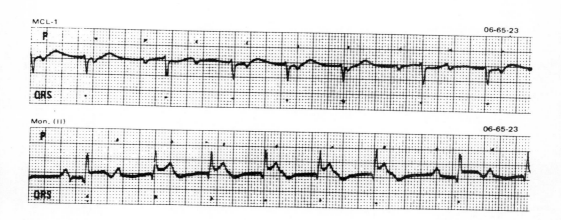

ANSWERS TO PROBLEMS—CHAPTER III

1. *ten*

2. $0.20{\overline{)60.00}}^{300}$

3. *0.12 and 0.20 sec.*

4. *0.10 sec.*

5. Rate *75/min.*

   PR *0.14 sec.*

   QRS *0.11 sec.*

6. *the number of 0.20 sec. squares between cycles.*

7. *208/min. Note the artifact due to standardization.*

ANSWERS TO PROBLEMS—CHAPTER IV

1. *toward*

2. *perpendicular*

3. *P*

4. *left leg.*

5. *positive*

6. *downward and to the left.*

ANSWERS TO PROBLEMS—CHAPTER V

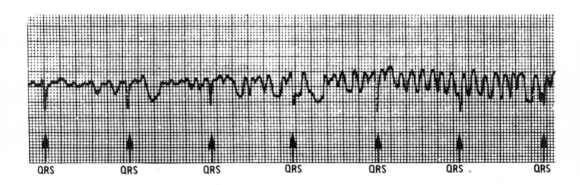

1. **QRS Complexes:** *Ventricular rate 56/min. QRS duration 0.06 sec. Ventricular rhythm regular.*

   Atrial Complexes: *P waves are obscured by jerky undulation of the baseline.*

   Conclusion: *An artifact of this regularity could not be due only to a loose electrode. Some regularly occurring motion must play a role. This patient had itchy skin; whenever he scratched near the electrode site, the rapid vibratory motion of skin and underlying muscles produced this pattern, resembling ventricular fibrillation.*

2. *technique.*

3.   *True   False*

   1. *X*

   2. *X*

   3. *X*

   4. *X*

ANSWERS TO PROBLEMS—CHAPTER VI

1. *Technique is satisfactory. Ventricular rhythm is regular at a rate of 58. QRS complexes are uniform, 0.05 sec. A-V conduction is slightly delayed, for the PR interval is 0.21 sec.*

   Conclusion: *Sinus bradycardia. Delay in atrio-ventricular conduction. (In Chapter XVI this will be called "first degree A-V block.")*

2. Conclusion: *Sinus rhythm with premature QRS complexes which are different from the QRS in sinus cycles. Rate 80/min. PR 0.14 sec. QRS 0.08 sec. Note that the rhythm of the sinus P waves is not upset by the interposed premature beats. The interval between b and d is just twice the standard P-P interval. Indeed, P wave c is recognized hiding in the T wave of QRS number three.*

3. *Sudden deflections of the baseline must be artifacts, probably due to movement of an electrode. QRS complexes are uniform, 0.08 sec. Ventricular rate about 60/min. PR 0.16 sec.*

   Conclusion: *Sinus rhythm. Wandering baseline.*

4. *The QRS complexes are uniform and broad, 0.14 sec. The rate is 50/min. A-V conduction is delayed. The PR interval is 0.23 sec.*

   Conclusion: *Sinus bradycardia. Conduction through the ventricles is slow. (In Chapter VIII this will be called "bundle branch block.")*

5. *After two sinus cycles at a rate of about 70/min., there is marked slowing. Cycles no. 3, 4 and 5 occur at a rate of 37/min. The rate then returns to about 70/min. Note the slight variation in P wave contour and PR interval.*

   Conclusion: *Sinus arrhythmia. PR 0.16–0.20 sec. QRS 0.07 sec.*

6. *Conclusion: Acceleration of the sinus rate after a period without ventricular response. Three P waves are not followed by QRS complexes.*

ANSWERS TO PROBLEMS—CHAPTER VII

1. *ectopic*

2. *sinus node*

3. *20–40/min.*

4. *automaticity*

5. *Enhanced automaticity*

6. *broad or narrow.*

7. *Strips A, D, and E have a narrow QRS and can only be supraventricular.*

   Strips B, C, F and G have a broad QRS and are either ventricular or supraventricular with abnormal ventricular conduction.

8. *Yes.*

   A regular ventricular rhythm is present at a rate of 168/min. This must be either (a) ventricular tachycardia or (b) supraventricular tachycardia with abnormal ventricular conduction. Atrial activity is not apparent.

ANSWERS TO PROBLEMS—CHAPTER VIII

1. *The QRS duration is normal in this lead. Multiple leads would be needed to determine if a different "point of view" (a different lead axis) would show the true QRS duration substantially longer, indicating bundle branch block.*

   Rhythm is not perfectly regular. Such variation is dignified by the term sinus arrhythmia when the P-P interval varies 10–15%. Also, a single VPC is present.

2. *Although QRS duration appears to be 0.09 sec. in lead II (the standard monitoring lead axis), the presence of bundle branch block is indicated by the configuration and duration shown in lead V2, 0.13 sec.*

3. *What appears to be depressed ST segment in lead II is shown in V6 to be part of QRS. Lead V6 indicates BBB with a QRS duration of 0.13 sec.*

4. *No. The diagnosis of bundle branch block can be made only if there is evidence of supraventricular origin. This requires that one be able to infer that QRS is due to P. In this case, in the top strip there is a regular*

ventricular rhythm at a rate of 38/min. and a regular atrial rhythm at a rate of about 92/min. Is QRS due to P? This seems unlikely since the PR interval is completely variable. (In Chapter XVI this will be described as complete or "third degree" A-V block.)

In the bottom strip, the broadness of complexes g, h, and i would not be attributed to bundle branch block unless there were some reason to believe they were initiated by a supraventricular focus.

ANSWERS TO PROBLEMS—CHAPTER IX

1. *Ventricular rhythm fundamentally is regular at a rate of 84/min. QRS duration is 0.09 sec. PR interval 0.17 sec.*

   The QRS complexes are uniform but the eighth complex is premature. Its appearance is about the same as in the sinus cycles; therefore it must be supraventricular in origin. Is it preceded by a premature P wave? Indeed it is, hidden in the ST-T of the previous cycle.

   Conclusion: *Sinus rhythm with one APC.*

2. *Sinus rhythm is interrupted by two premature complexes with a configuration only slightly different from that of the sinus cycles. Because they so nearly resemble the sinus beats, we suspect supraventricular origin and look particularly closely for a preceding premature P. Note distortion of the T waves preceding each premature beat. Each premature QRS is preceded by a premature P which is hidden in the T of the preceding cycle.*

   Conclusion: *Sinus rhythm. Rate 83/min. PR 0.18 sec. QRS 0.08 sec. Two APC's with slightly abnormal (aberrant) ventricular conduction.*

3. *Recognizing that the premature QRS is narrow and the same as in the sinus cycles, we know it is of supraventricular origin. There are only two types of supraventricular premature beats—atrial and junctional.*

   Is it preceded by an upright premature P? It is. This settles the question. The premature QRS is due to an APC.

4. *The discussion of question 3 also applies here.*

5. *Bigeminal rhythm is present. It seems fair to assume that the first in each pair (No. 1, 3, 5, 7 and 9) is a sinus cycle. Origin of the second cycle in each pair is the remaining question. Each (No. 2, 4, 6, 8 and 10) is preceded by a sharp negative deflection, a premature P. Various degrees*

of aberration account for variable configuration of the QRS complexes which occur in response to the coupled APC's.

6. *Regular rhythm is interrupted by a premature QRS which is "different" but not preceded by a premature P. A negative P comes immediately afterward, indicating junctional origin with retrograde depolarization of the atria. The altered QRS configuration must be due to altered conduction within the ventricles, an illustration of abnormal (aberrant) ventricular conduction.*

How is it possible for QRS to precede P when the rhythm is initiated above the ventricles? The ladder diagram is useful. (Note that depolarization of the A-V node produces no deflection on the usual ECG).

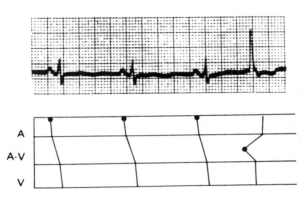

Possibly the depolarization wave is initiated in the lower portion of the junctional tissue. It promptly reaches the rapidly conducting His-Purkinje system and soon is transmitted throughout the ventricle, producing the QRS.

Meanwhile, laboriously it is making its way upward.

Eventually it breaks out of the junctional tissue and spreads rapidly through the atria. Since atrial depolarization occurs in a headward direction, the P wave is inverted in the monitoring lead with negative electrode at the right shoulder.

Conclusion: *Junctional premature complex with prior activation of the ventricles and aberrant ventricular conduction.*

7. *These regularly occurring QRS complexes are not preceded by P waves. Instead, the P comes immediately afterward and is inverted.*

Conclusion: *Junctional rhythm with prior activation of the ventricles.*

8. *One premature QRS interrupts sinus rhythm. The premature QRS is a bit "different." It is not preceded by a premature P. There is, however, an inverted P immediately following it, indicating junctional origin. (See discussion of question 6.)*

9.

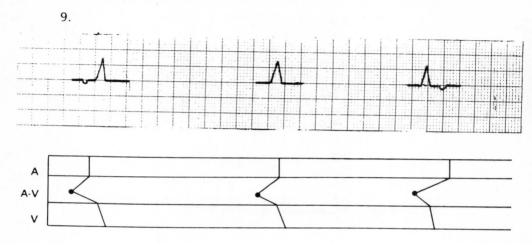

10. *Ventricular rhythm is irregular due to premature complexes No. 3, 5 and 7. When confronted with a premature QRS, proceed through a standard inquiry to determine if it is of ventricular or supraventricular origin.*

   Cycle No. 7 is premature, narrow and about the same as the dominant QRS pattern. This alone identifies its supraventricular origin, confirmed by the premature P, hidden in the T wave of cycle No. 6, and the less-than-compensatory pause.

   Cycles No. 3 and 5 are broad and "different." A premature QRS which is anomalous may be either ventricular or supraventricular with aberrant ventricular conduction.

   Each is followed by a pause which is less than compensatory, and each is preceded by a premature P. Note the importance of inspecting the T wave which precedes a premature QRS cycle. Could the T be distorted by a premature P? Note how the T of cycle No. 4 differs from the T of cycles No. 1 and 8.

   Conclusion: *Sinus rhythm, rate 72/min. QRS 0.05 sec. PR 0.16 sec. Several APC's, two of which are associated with aberrant ventricular conduction.*

11. *The premature complexes, though broad and "different," are preceded by premature P waves—distorting the prior T waves. APC's usually do not respond to lidocaine.*

ANSWERS TO PROBLEMS—CHAPTER X

1. 1. *"different"*
   2. *suddenly*
   3. *sudden*
   4. *constant*
   5. *no effect or it stops the paroxysm.*

2.

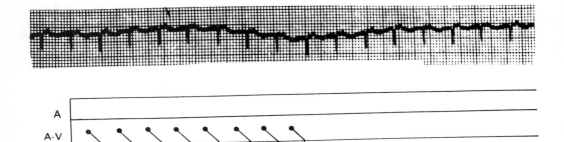

ANSWERS TO PROBLEMS—CHAPTER XI

1. *Atrial rate is 300/min. The diagnosis is atrial flutter.*

2.

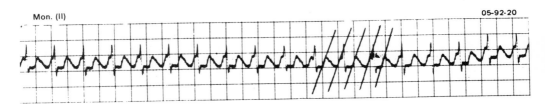

1. *330/min.*
2. *165/min.*
3. *2:1*

3. 1. *84/min.*
   2. *360/min.*
   3. *II—No*
      V1—Yes
   4. *Atrial flutter with variable block.*

4. 1. *atrial flutter with 2:1 block.*
   2. *aberrant*
   3. *impairs*
   4. *94/min.*
      262/min.

5. 1. *Ventricular rate 134/min. Ventricular rhythm regular.*
   2. *"Always think of ATRIAL FLUTTER WITH 2:1 BLOCK."*
   3. *"COULD ANOTHER P WAVE BE HIDDEN HALFWAY BETWEEN THE OBVIOUS P WAVES?"*
   4. *0.46 sec.*
      0.23 sec.
      Yes.
   5. *Carotid sinus massage.*
      Additional leads.
   6. *True.*
   7. *Atrial rate 280/min. Atrial rhythm regular. Rhythm diagnosis: atrial flutter.*
   8. *Digitalis might slow the ventricular rate but it is notoriously unreliable in the sick patient with flutter. Cardioversion is the recommended treatment in this patient who steadily is getting worse.*
   9. *Following cardioversion, sinus rhythm has appeared.*

ANSWERS TO PROBLEMS—CHAPTER XII

1. A. *irregular.*
      flutter.
   B. *probably prolonged, 0.12 sec.*
      probably supraventricular, because QRS configuration same as one minute earlier, tracing A.
      probably junctional, with simultaneous depolarization of atria and ventricles.
   C. *sinus*
   D. *fibrillation*
      240/min.
      flutter waves
      atrial flutter

2. A. *supraventricular*
   B. *irregular*
   C. *slight*
   D. *absent*
   E. *absent*
   F. *atrial fibrillation*

3. A. *totally irregular*
   B. *a likely diagnosis*

4. *atrial fibrillation*

5. Ventricular Complexes: *Two families of QRS complexes are present. Further, the QRS complexes occur in couplets. The first of each pair is narrow (0.07 sec.). The second is broad (0.13 sec.).*

   Ventricular rhythm is irregular but not completely so. The R-R is uniform within each pair, numbers 1–2, 3–4, 5–6, 7–8. Each of these R-R intervals equals 0.60 sec. Further, R-R intervals 3–5, 5–7 are equal (1.72 sec.).

   Atrial Complexes: *The small amplitude undulations between No. 2 and 3 are suggestive of fibrillation waves. Perhaps a chest lead would demonstrate them better.*

   Conclusion: *Atrial fibrillation with a slow ventricular rate suggests digitalis effect. Further, the pronounced slowing with coupled ectopic beats suggest digitalis excess. The regularization of QRS complexes also indicates a high degree of A-V block with escape of a junctional pacemaker (No. 3, 5 and 7). These findings indicate the probability of digitalis poisoning.*

6. *This is too regular for atrial fibrillation; several R-R intervals are exactly the same, 0.42 sec. The rhythm is atrial flutter with variable block. At first glance, an atrial rate of 150 might be considered. However, remember the rule: "Divide the obvious P-P interval in half and ask: 'Could another P wave be hidden halfway between the obvious P waves?' " Here, note that the atrial rate actually is 300/min.*

   Discussion: *A fast ventricular rate means a short diastolic period. Diastole occurs between the end of the T wave and the beginning of the next QRS complex. It is during this period that the ventricles have an opportunity to rest and during which they are filled. A fast rate therefore may lead to inefficient pumping. Digitalis slows the ventricular rate in atrial flutter and fibrillation by producing a certain amount of A-V block, decreasing the number of "f" waves which the junctional tissue can conduct.*

7. *Probably not. The underlying rhythm is atrial fibrillation. The rhythm of the anomalous cycles is irregular. The initial QRS vector is not disturbed. Probably they represent aberration rather than ventricular ectopy. (Remember: With aberration, an RSR' pattern in MCL-1 is usual, not invariable.)*

ANSWERS TO PROBLEMS—CHAPTER XIII

1. *Cycles d and g are premature. These QRS complexes are broad and "different." They are not preceded by a premature P wave. However, they do seem to interrupt the atrial rhythm; the interval between cycles f and h is not exactly twice the interval between cycles e and f. The interval between cycles b and c is 0.96 sec. Therefore, one might expect cycle e to occur 1.92 (0.96 $\times$ 2) sec. after cycle c. In actuality, cycle e occurs 1.84 sec. after cycle c. It is worth remembering that the pause after a VPC often is not precisely "compensatory." Sinus arrhythmia is the common explanation, but always consider retrograde conduction when a VPC seems to upset the atrial rhythm.*

   QRS Complexes: *Not uniform; the premature cycles are broad and "different."*

   Conclusion: *Sinus rhythm is interrupted by two VPC's.*

   Clinical Commentary: *During the early days after myocardial infarction, VPC's may warn of impending ventricular tachycardia or fibrillation. Lidocaine is the most commonly used drug.*

2. *The VPC's are frequent, multiform and have a variable coupling interval. They cannot be attributed to sinus bradycardia for careful search indicates the atrial rate is 76/min., not 38/min. P waves e, f and g give the true P-P interval, 0.78 sec.*

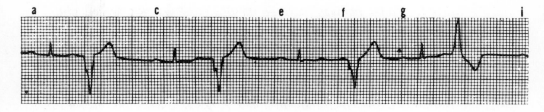

   Atrial rate is significant when considering VPC's, for bradycardia facilitates ectopic activity. A simplistic explanation is as follows:

   The faster the rate, the greater proportion of time the ventricles are refractory.

3. *Yes. There is a pair, and the VPC's are frequent and of variable configuration.*

4. *Yes, two of these VPC's occur on the T·wave, and are likely to trigger repetitive ectopic beats, ventricular tachycardia or fibrillation.*

5. *Sinus P waves occur at a rate of 55/min. Each sinus cycle is followed by a broad and different QRS, an example of bigeminy due to VPC's. Note the inverted P after each QRS, an example of retrograde conduction to the atria.*

6. *Ventricular rhythm is nearly regular, about 150/min. Atrial flutter is likely. The broad and different QRS complexes are not really premature and probably represent aberrant ventricular conduction.*

ANSWERS TO PROBLEMS—CHAPTER XIV

1. *The underlying rhythm is sinus, with a ventricular rate of 70/min. QRS duration is 0.07 sec. Several clues suggest that the bouts of "broad QRS tachycardia" are ventricular in origin:*

    1. *This clinical setting is one often associated with ventricular arrhythmias.*
    2. *Although we do not see independent atrial activity during the paroxysm, the bouts do not interrupt atrial rhythm; the P waves come about at the expected time.*
    3. *The initial beat of the paroxysm is not preceded by a premature P and thus has earmarks of a VPC.*

2. *Broad QRS complexes are present at a rate of 168/min. and the ventricular rhythm is regular; in fact it is precisely regular. Precise regularity is said to favor a supraventricular origin. If prompt treatment were indicated, no doubt we would proceed on the assumption this represents ventricular tachycardia, knowing full well this could be supraventricular with abnormal ventricular conduction.*

3. 1. *It would be helpful to know the response to carotid sinus pressure. If supraventricular, the tachycardia might be terminated; or enhanced A-V block from vagal stimulation might slow the QRS complexes, revealing underlying atrial tachycardia with 1:1 conduction, or atrial flutter with 2:1 conduction.*
    2. *The clinical setting. Is this a patient with recent infarction, or is it a young woman with a long history of bouts of tachycardia of sudden onset and cessation?*
    3. *Has the tachycardia been preceded by clearcut VPC's, occurring singly and in clusters?*
    4. *Get additional leads which are likely to improve chances of seeing P waves and thus demonstrate unrelated atrial activity. If a twelve lead tracing does not suffice, additional V leads on the right chest may help. Otherwise, an atrial electrogram is the next diagnostic step. However,*

in the CCU most such patients will be treated promptly with a pre-sumptive diagnosis of ventricular tachycardia.

4. A) *Assuming the P-P interval is 1.0 sec., the tachycardia could be dia-grammed as follows:*

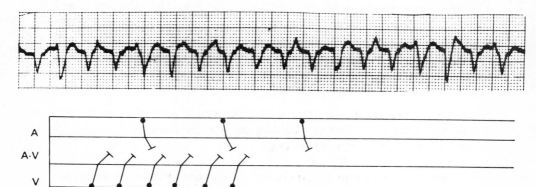

B) *Assuming the P-P interval is 0.5 sec., the tachycardia could be dia-grammed as follows:*

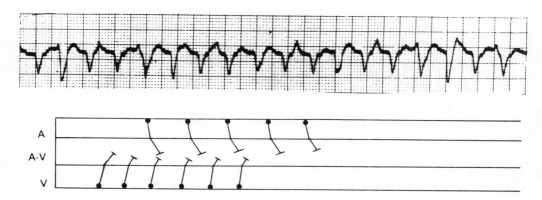

C) *With either hypothesis, the probable diagnosis is ventricular tachy-cardia.*

5. A) *Assuming the P-P interval is 1.84 sec., the arrhythmia could be diagrammed as follows:*

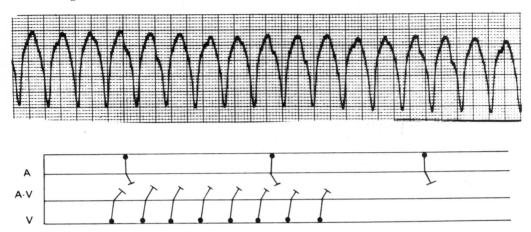

B) *An alternate hypothesis could be diagrammed as follows:*

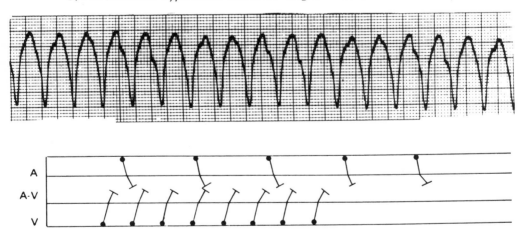

6. *Ventricular rate 188/min.*

QRS duration 0.12 sec.

The rhythm is quite regular, probably precisely regular.

Independent atrial activity is not seen.

Conclusion: *This is either ventricular tachycardia or supraventricular tachycardia with aberrant ventricular conduction. As usual, a firm distinc-*

tion is not possible. The ventricular rate is too slow for atrial flutter with 1:1 conduction, too fast for atrial flutter with 2:1 conduction.

7. *Treatment, however, presents no problem. If a thump on the precordium is not curative, precordial shock is essential and cannot be delayed in this patient who is dying from the effects of tachycardia.*

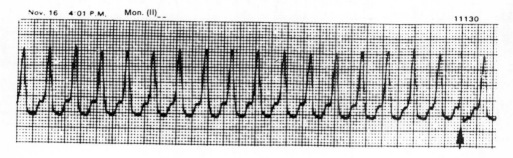

Nov. 16   4·01 P.M.   Mon. (II)   11130

Note how much additional help is available from the longer strip. A Dressler beat is shown. This indicates independent atrial activity and nearly clinches the diagnosis of ventricular tachycardia.

ANSWERS TO PROBLEMS—CHAPTER XV

1. *ventricular fibrillation.*

2. *precordial shock.*

3. *chest compression.*

4. *ventricular fibrillation.*

5. *precordial shock*

6. *Initially the rhythm is slow and regular, 45/min. QRS is broad and not preceded by P, probably an ectopic escape mechanism. Ventricular fibrillation develops after a VPC.*

ANSWERS TO PROBLEMS—CHAPTER XVI

1. *Slight wandering baseline.*

   Regular ventricular rhythm at a rate of 60/min. QRS duration about 0.10 sec. There is just enough variation in configuration to raise a question regarding alteration in intraventricular conduction. The cyclic nature of the change together with the wandering baseline, however, suggest respiratory change in heart position relative to the monitoring lead axis.

The PR interval varies from 0.20 to 0.24 sec. We do not know what this variation means. Each P is followed by a QRS.

Conclusion: *First degree A-V heart block.*

Clinical Commentary: *Sinus bradycardia with a prolonged PR interval is a characteristic combination during the early hours after posterior infarction. The artery which supplies the posterior portion of the heart also sends branches to the A-V node and sinus node. When A-V conduction is slightly delayed in patients with recent infarction, it is advisable to observe closely for development of a higher degree of A-V block.*

2. *Orthopnea, hypotension, fever and a high SGOT level all indicate substantial pump damage. No doubt stroke volume is quite low.*

3. *Probably nothing. Digitalis, Isuprel, Glucagon, Ephedrine, or Dopamine might be considered.*

4.

Cardiac output = Stroke volume $\times$ Heart rate

Following infarction, stroke volume is low and fixed. Thus the best route to a better cardiac output is increased heart rate for this patient with an inappropriately slow rate of 60/min. Atropine or pacing would be useful.

5. *Ventricular rhythm is irregular. QRS configuration varies but the odd beats are not premature. In fact, they occur with a smaller R-R interval than in the narrower complexes which are preceded by P waves. QRS duration is variable. In those cycles preceded by a P with a PR interval of about 0.20 sec., QRS duration is 0.10 sec.; elsewhere it is wider. The third QRS in the second strip may be a fusion beat.*

P waves are fairly regular at a rate of 58/min. The fourth P is not conducted and the fifth occurs so soon after a QRS we are not surprised that it is not conducted. It occurs when the ventricles are refractory.

PR interval is 0.20 sec. in the majority of the sinus cycles. The fourth, fifth, sixth and ninth P waves are not conducted. It is in this portion of the record that the broad, "different" QRS complexes occur.

Conclusion: *Second degree A-V heart block. Ventricular escape beats. Fusion beat.*

Clinical Commentary: *Ectopic ventricular beats which develop in response to A-V block ordinarily should not be treated with depressant drugs such as Xylocaine, quinidine or Pronestyl; death may result from suppression of the life-saving ectopic mechanism.*

6. *Rapid, uniform deflections characteristic of ventricular flutter terminate spontaneously and are followed by bradycardia of ectopic atrial origin.*

Clinical Commentary: *Ventricular flutter usually progresses to ventricular fibrillation. During ventricular flutter, mechanical activity of the heart is absent, circulation ceases and death commonly results. However, brief episodes of ventricular flutter may be responsible for Adams-Stokes syncopal attacks. Adams-Stokes syncope also may result from bradycardia or tachysystole.*

7. *Features of ventricular tachycardia gradually change to uniform, smooth undulations characteristic of ventricular flutter.*

8. *Irregular undulations without recognizable QRS indicate ventricular fibrillation. Towards the end of the top strip, there is an instrumental artifact due to precordial shock. After defibrillation there is a slow supraventricular mechanism with broad, bizarre QRS complexes.*

9. *A pacing catheter was inserted.*

Discussion: *When there are two families of QRS complexes it is worthwhile to consider them individually. Here, the narrow sort are preceded by P waves with a PR interval of 0.24 sec. Atrial activity then continues without interruption but the remaining QRS complexes are broad, perfectly regular and introduced by the characteristic pacemaker artifact.*

The pacemaker was turned on after two normal sinus cycles. (Note the similarity between the first two cycles in the strip and the tracing shown in question 5.)

10. *Each QRS is preceded by a P wave. Atrial rhythm is regular but PR progressively lengthens. After the non-conducted P, PR is shorter. This is the Wenckebach variety of second degree A-V block.*

11. *regular.*

12. *regular.*

13. *variable.*

14. *3°*

15. *junctional tissue*

16. *40–60/min.*

17. *transient*

18. *superiorly and to the left.*

19. *anterior*

index